PHLEBOTOMY
BEST PRACTICES

A CASE STUDY APPROACH

PHLEBOTOMY BEST PRACTICES

A CASE STUDY APPROACH

Carol Itatani, PhD, MS, MT (ASCP), PBT (ASCP)

California State University at Long Beach
Professor
Biological Sciences

Norma Shipp, MS, MT (ASCP), PBT

St. Mary Medical Center, Laboratory
Long Beach, CA
POC and Phlebotomy Coordinator
Professor
Biological Sciences

Lippincott Williams & Wilkins
a Wolters Kluwer business
Philadelphia · Baltimore · New York · London
Buenos Aires · Hong Kong · Sydney · Tokyo

Acquisitions Editor: Peter Sabatini
Managing Editor: Kevin C. Dietz
Marketing Manager: Allison M. Noplock
Production Editor: Sirkka Bertling
Design Coordinator: Holly Reid McLaughlin
Compositor: International Typesetting and Composition
Printer: Data Reproductions Corporation

Library of Congress Cataloging-in-Publication Data

Itatani, Carol Ann.
   Phlebotomy best practices : a case study approach / Carol Itatani, Norma Shipp.
     p. cm.
   Includes bibliographical references and index.
   ISBN-13:   978-0-7817-7731-5
   ISBN-10:   0-7817-7731-3
  1.   Phlebotomy—Decision making—Case studies. 2.   Phlebotomy—Decision making—Problems, exercises, etc. 3.   Problem-based learning. I. Shipp, Norma. II. Title.

   RB45.15.I83 2006
   616.07′561—dc22   2006017279

To purchase additional copies of this book, call our customer service department at **(800) 638-3030** or fax orders to **(301) 223-2320.** International customers should call **(301) 223-2300.**

Visit Lippincott Williams & Wilkins on the Internet: http://www.LWW.com. Lippincott Williams & Wilkins customer service representatives are available from 8:30 am to 6:00 pm, EST.

06 07 08 09 10
1 2 3 4 5 6 7 8 9 10

Preface

Phlebotomy is a dynamic and important medical profession. You as the phlebotomist have direct contact with the patient and are the face, the representative of the Clinical Laboratory. Your skills and professional behavior greatly influence the patient's opinions and attitudes about the quality of the health care they are receiving. Therefore, this book of case studies was designed specifically to help you apply the information you are learning as new phlebotomists, or to help you as a veteran phlebotomist to review and enhance your background information. Our objective in writing this book is to ensure that the person (you) who is obtaining the patient's blood is *truly* a medical professional.

To use this book most effectively, read a case and then compose answers to each of the questions that follow the case. Each of the cases can be used for individual instruction, or to make learning and review more fun and interesting; these cases can also be discussed with a couple of friends or colleagues. Once you have composed answers to each question, turn to the discussion of each case. The discussion provides answers, and in many cases, further information to explain *why* a procedure is performed a certain way, *why* it is important to pay attention to this detail, or *what* the consequences are of mistakes and errors in phlebotomy.

After reading and digesting the information provided in the discussion, go back to the Key Words listed at the beginning of each case. Quiz yourself on their meanings. Do you know what each term means? Can you explain these terms to someone else? If you can do this, congratulations! You have successfully completed the case study and now know how to professionally and ethically respond in a similar situation.

Cases are loosely organized by a common topic into chapters. We have tried to tie cases together according to major problems faced in the everyday work environment of phlebotomists. Pay attention to chapter titles to identify the common thread linking these cases. For further review and to ensure full understanding of the issues involved in each chapter, a chapter quiz is provided. Objective questions are easy! Most of these questions ask you to recognize terms and test your recall of details. A better way to test your understanding is to answer the essay questions. We recommend writing a paragraph or two. Essay questions ask you to explain, describe, and apply information. If you can provide complete answers to essay questions, you are knowledgeable about this topic. You know your stuff, and are a competent, professional phlebotomist.

Best Wishes in Your Chosen Career,

Carol Itatani and Norma Shipp

Instructors of phlebotomy courses will find this book of case studies a great way to enhance your course materials and teaching techniques. Furthermore, an instructor's guide with teaching tips and best practices in the classroom is available at: http://connection.lww.com/Itatani should you decide to adopt this book.

Table of Contents

Site Selection and Risk Factors

CASE 1
Optimal Site for "Stat" Glucose

Patient A.K., a 65-year-old white woman, is hospitalized for a broken arm and has a cast on the left arm. The right arm has an IV drip running. The patient is a diabetic who needs a glucose determination "stat."

Key Words: dermal puncture • diabetes • edema • glucometer • point-of-care instrumentation (POC) • stat

QUESTIONS

1. What is the optimal site for phlebotomy?
2. Why were other sites rejected?
3. What is the optimal procedure for obtaining the blood sample?
4. How does the designation "stat" influence the procedure?

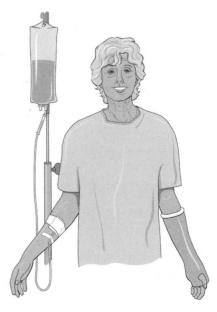

Figure 1.1. Pateint With Both Arms Unavailable.

DISCUSSION OF CASE STUDY

1. Neither of this patient's arms can be used for venipuncture in the ante-cubital area. The left arm has a cast, and the right arm has an intravenous (IV) drip "running." The antecubital area of the right arm might be accessible, but it is not an appropriate site because the venous blood in that area will be diluted by the IV (Fig. 1.1).

2. The patient's legs and feet are not an option because the patient is diabetic. Diabetics often have poor circulation in the lower extremities and are more vulnerable to infection.

   Diabetes is a metabolic endocrine disorder that is becoming more common with increasing obesity among the US population. Type I diabetes is a deficiency of the hormone insulin and occurs more commonly among children. Type II diabetes is also called adult-onset and occurs more commonly among older adults. In type II diabetes, varying degrees of insulin deficiency occur, but also insulin resistance. Cells in the body do not utilize insulin, and as a result, cells do not utilize glucose (blood sugar) efficiently. Glucose therefore accumulates in the blood and in other tissues and is the cause of many other disease complications.

3. A finger-stick is the optimal procedure for obtaining the blood sample. The third or fourth finger of the right hand is probably the most useful site. Fingers of the left hand may be edematous (swollen) because of the fracture on that side. If fingers of the right hand are edematous because of a previous IV localized near this site, the blood specimen could theoretically be drawn below the IV. The recommended procedure is to stop the current IV for 2 minutes and perform a venipuncture below the IV, possibly from a hand vein. Experience has shown that specimens are not always acceptable if drawn below the IV while the IV is on. The phlebotomist should indicate on the specimen tube that the blood was drawn below the IV.

   Edema of the fingers may contribute excess tissue fluids to the blood sample and potentially dilute the capillary blood sample, thus lowering the blood glucose level.

4. This order is a stat, which indicates that results need to be determined instantly or as rapidly as possible. A glucose determination can be performed using a glucometer (point-of-care) instrument. This instrument can provide glucose levels very rapidly at the bedside. Point-of-care devices were developed for this type of situation. The results are immediate, and the patient can be treated quickly.

CASE 2
Mastectomy

Mrs. S.J., a 75-year-old white woman, comes into the oncology clinic for her annual check-up. After visiting with her doctor, she is sent to the laboratory for a complete blood count (CBC), liver panel, and erythrocyte sedimentation rate (ESR). Susan, the phlebotomist, correctly identifies

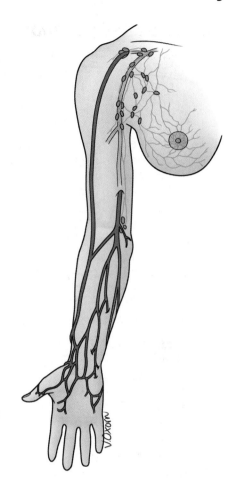

Figure 1.2. Superficial venous and lymphatic drainage of the upper limb. Anterior view of the upper limb showing the cephalic and basilic veins and their tributaries. (Reprinted with permission from Moore KL, Agur A. Essential Clinical Anatomy. 2nd Ed. Philadelphia: Lippincott Williams & Wilkins, 2002.)

the patient, preps the site, gathers appropriate equipment and supplies, and asks from which arm Mrs. S.J. prefers to have her blood drawn. Mrs. S.J. tells Susan that she had a mastectomy 3 years ago on the left side and most of the time has blood drawn from the right (Fig. 1.2).

Key Words: mastectomy • metastatic • lymphostasis

QUESTIONS

   1. Which arm should Susan use for obtaining the blood sample?

   2. Does the mastectomy make a difference? Why?

   3. Does the length of time since the mastectomy make a difference?

   4. What tubes do you need for the tests ordered? In what order do you draw the blood if using a Vacutainer?

DISCUSSION OF CASE STUDY

   1. Susan should use Mrs. S.J.'s right arm for obtaining the blood sample.

   2. A mastectomy definitely makes a difference in selection of the appropriate arm for venipuncture. If a woman has breast cancer, not only is

the cancer removed, but also the lymph nodes from the adjacent axillary (armpit) area are removed and examined to determine whether the cancer has spread. Lymph nodes are tiny filtering units and are the first place that metastatic (breakaway) breast cancer cells may be found. Therefore, the mastectomy patient may have lymphostasis because of the removal of lymph tissue. Lymphostasis can result in failure or inhibition of lymph fluid movement, making the patient more susceptible to infection. Tourniquet pressure could also cause harm to the arm and pain for the patient.

3. Generally, the length of time since a mastectomy was performed will not make a difference. Each patient is different, and only his or her physician can determine what if any blood collection can be performed.

4. For the liver panel, use a light green-top or dark green-top (lithium heparin) tube. Some laboratories require a red-top or gold-top tube for a liver panel, depending on the type of clinical chemistry instrumentation being used. The CBC requires a lavender-top tube. The ESR can be performed on the same tube drawn for the CBC. Some ESR procedures require a black-top tube, which contains sodium citrate.

    Order of draw using a Vacutainer would be green, black, and/or lavender tops. If the liver panel requires serum, then the red-top or gold-top tube is drawn first.

CASE 3
Burn Patient

Patient J.T., a 45-year-old black man, was hospitalized for severe burns on both arms. To provide adequate hydration, the patient has a central venous catheter (CVC). Legs and feet are not accessible for blood collection because they are reserving these areas for possible autologous skin transplant. A CBC and electrolytes have been ordered for this patient.

Key Words: allogeneic • autologous • AV (arterial venous) shunt • central venous catheter (CVC) • heparin or saline lock • implanted port • PICC line • vascular access devices

QUESTIONS

1. Where would you obtain a blood sample from this patient?

2. Into what veins is a CVC generally implanted? Is this site accessible? What precautions should be taken?

3. What does autologous mean?

4. What is the minimum amount of blood needed for these tests?

DISCUSSION OF CASE STUDY

1. The blood sample must be obtained from the CVC line. However, only properly trained personnel should draw blood from CVC lines. Phlebotomists should give the tubes to the person who is drawing the specimen or stand by to receive the blood specimen in a syringe to transfer to appropriate tubes. The nursing staff may refer to CVC lines by different names, which include Broviac, Groshong, Hickman, and triple-lumen (Fig. 1.3).

2. The CVC line is inserted into the subclavian vein and advanced into the superior vena caval vein proximal to the right atrium. Because this is an access tube inserted directly into the central blood circulation, only properly trained personnel should draw blood from CVC lines. Lines must be flushed properly to prevent coagulation and plugging of the line. The right amount of pressure must be applied to retrieve a specimen without collapsing the line, and care must be taken not to dislodge or introduce any contamination into the line. Phlebotomists should give the tubes to the health care professional drawing the blood sample or stand by to receive the specimen in a syringe to be transferred to the proper tubes. Because these vascular access devices (VADs) are often flushed with saline or heparin, the first sample of blood collected through the device should not be used. The amount of blood discarded depends on the type of VAD, the amount of dead space in the line, and the blood tests to be performed. For routine blood tests, usually a 5-mL discard sample is sufficient. Coagulation testing may require a larger amount of blood to be discarded. The phlebotomist needs to indicate on the blood tubes that blood was drawn from a VAD. Review in your phlebotomy manual for PICC line, AV (arterial venous) shunt, heparin, or saline lock and implanted port.

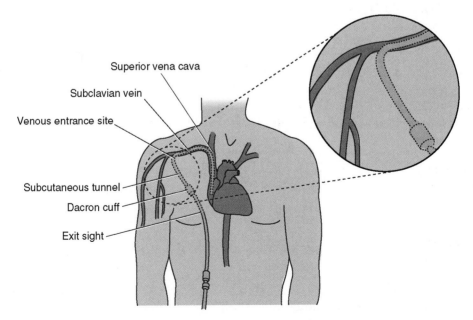

Figure 1.3. Central venous catheter (CVC). (Reprinted with permission from McCall RE, Tankersley CM. Phlebotomy Essentials. 3rd Ed. Philadelphia: Lippincott Williams & Wilkins, 2003.)

3. Autologous means self. Autologous donation is the process by which a person can donate his/her own blood, or in this case skin, for his/her own use. Skin is removed from one part of the body and donated to another part of the body needing new skin. Because this is the patient's own skin, there is no tissue rejection to worry about. Tissue that is donated and transplanted from another person is referred to as an allograft or an allogenic graft. Because every individual has antigens unique to his or her own cells, allograft rejection of tissue is a problem. Examples of allografts include blood transfusions, kidney, or bone marrow transplants.

4. Because this patient will need long-term follow-up, minimal amounts of blood should be drawn. The minimum amount of blood needed for these tests is 0.5 mL for the CBC and 0.8 to 1.0 mL for electrolytes. Most chemistry instruments need 0.25 to 0.5 mL serum or plasma to run a test. If filling a Microtainer tube with venous blood, indicate on the tube that blood was drawn from a vein. Microtainer specimens are generally capillary blood. Normal reference ranges for test results can vary between capillary and venous blood samples. Thus, indicate the source.

CASE 4
2-Year-Old Child

Patient C.M. is a 2-year-old white girl who needs a CBC, lead, and antibody test for measles, mumps, and rubella (MMR). The child is fearful and crying, and the teenage mother is not in much better shape. A blood drawing room for children is available. Penny is the phlebotomist available for drawing this child.

Key Words: lead determinations • MMR vaccination and antibody response • pediatric venipuncture • restraint methods

QUESTIONS

1. How should Penny calm the mother and child?

2. How should Penny restrain the child?

3. Where should she obtain the blood sample? What is the preferred site? Which method is preferred?

4. What equipment and tubes are necessary?

DISCUSSION OF CASE STUDY

1. Penny should present a professional appearance and a calm, confident, caring attitude. She may or may not want to wear a white coat. The white coat enhances her professional appearance, but it may also scare the child. Her confident actions will help gain the confidence of the child and the mother and relieve some of their fearfulness. A room specifically for children will help to present a comfortable environment.

- Have equipment ready to use before approaching the child.
- Explain to the parent and child what will be involved in the procedure. Explain to the child in language appropriate for her age. It also helps to talk to the child at his or her level. Sit or squat so that you can look her in the eye. Looming above her will make her more fearful.
- Involve the child; let the child select the arm or finger when appropriate.
- Let the child know that it will hurt at little. Be honest with children.
- Distract the child for the initial puncture and let the child know how long the draw will last.
- When the procedure is completed, praise and reward the child. Funny stickers, a happy face on the band-aid, or a blown-up latex glove can bring a smile and perhaps help make the next time less traumatic.

Excessive crying and stress can influence test results. The white blood cell (WBC) number in the CBC may become falsely elevated. If endocrine hormone levels were ordered, these test results could also be elevated. Therefore, to avoid emotional trauma for all participants and ensure test result accuracy, it is important to use communication skills effectively.

2. Immobilization or restraining the child during the procedure may be necessary to ensure his or her safety and yours (Fig. 1.4).

- Older children may be sitting on the parent's lap with the parent hugging the child and restraining the limb not being used. Penny should explain to the teenage mother that it would be helpful if she could

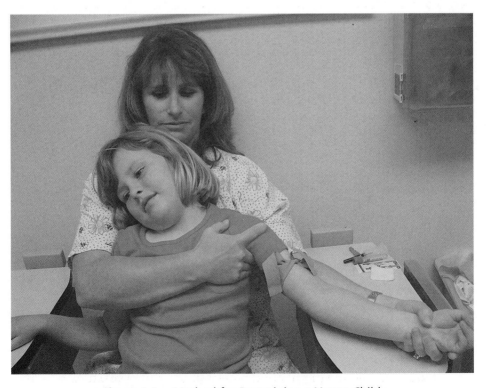

Figure 1.4. Method for Restraining a Young Child.

hold the child. If she seems very uncomfortable and fearful about doing this, it may be better if she does not remain in the room and another phlebotomist is called to help.

- Some children may need to be placed on a bed or drawing table lying down. A parent can rest his or her arm and body over the unused arm and legs to restrain the child.

  - If a parent or assistant is unavailable, a child can be restrained on a papoose board. Infants can be restrained by wrapping them up in a receiving blanket.

3. The preferred site for a 2-year-old child would be a finger-stick dermal puncture, if enough blood could be obtained for the requested test. Since over 4 mL of blood will be needed for the above tests, a syringe venous draw in the antecubital area would be recommended.

4. To perform a venous draw on a child this small, Penny should use a 23-gauge butterfly with a 5-mL syringe connected or pediatric-size Vacutainer tubes. The CBC will require 0.5 to 1.0 mL in a lavender-top tube, the antibody test will require 2.5 to 3.0 mL in a red-top tube, and the lead test will require 1.0 mL in a royal blue-top or brown-top tube. The order of draw for a Vacutainer would be red, royal blue, and lavender tops. If using a syringe, the order is reversed. Minimum blood volume may vary with the method and instrumentation used by a laboratory.

   Rubella is German measles. Most infants should receive their initial MMR vaccination at about 1 year of age. The vaccine consists of live, attenuated (weakened virus) vaccine, which will not cause disease. In response to vaccination, the immune system makes specific proteins called antibodies that will neutralize any exposure to pathogenic virus and thus prevent infectious disease. Antibodies can be detected in the serum and the amount of antibody measured to determine whether the child has been vaccinated and whether a good antibody response has occurred.

   Lead is a dangerous environmental contaminant, especially for children, because high levels will cause anemia and mental retardation. The royal blue tube has been specially formulated to contain very low levels of trace elements so that no interference will occur in measuring the amount of lead in the blood sample.

CASE 5
Obese Patient

Mrs. L.M. is a 58-year-old black woman who is very overweight (5'6", 250 lb). Her doctor has ordered thyroid tests, T3, T4, a liver panel, cholesterol, and triglycerides. She walked from the multilevel parking structure to the blood drawing center and is now experiencing a rapid heart beat and "lightheadedness." Mrs. L.M. informed Alejandro, the phlebotomist, that about an hour earlier the nurse in the doctor's office told her that her blood pressure was 160/95. Alejandro's initial venipuncture attempt was unsuccessful. On the second try, the patient complained of a sharp tingling pain at the site of venipuncture.

Key Words: fasting • hypertension • blood pressure • fainting • nerve damage

QUESTIONS

1. What should have been Alejandro's initial assessment of the patient?

2. How is a blood pressure of 160/95 interpreted? What do these numbers mean?

3. What tubes are necessary for the tests ordered? What anticoagulants are needed? Are there special transport conditions to be followed?

4. What procedures might have helped in obtaining the blood sample?

5. What complication occurred with the second attempt? What does Alejandro need to do now?

DISCUSSION OF CASE STUDY

1. Alejandro should have used his verbal and nonverbal skills to assess the patient. There are two issues that need to be addressed before drawing Mrs. L.M.'s blood sample. The first issue is whether Mrs. L.M. is fasting, and the second issue is her symptom of lightheadedness, which is a definite concern because she could faint.

   a. The triglyceride test requires a fasting specimen. Has the patient been fasting? If so, her lightheadedness may be because of low blood glucose. If she is diabetic and is taking diabetes medication, low blood sugar and fainting are even greater possibilities. If the patient has recently eaten, the blood should not be drawn at this time.

   b. Lightheadedness and a rapid heart beat may also be caused by overexertion. The patient should lie down or sit at rest until the symptoms disappear. This patient could potentially faint.

   Alejandro should ask Mrs. L.M. if she feels faint, if she has a history of fainting, and if so, would she like to lie down while having her blood drawn. This usually eliminates a fainting episode. Or if Mrs. L.M. does faint, then she is in a secure position.

   Should Mrs. L.M. decide not to lie down and then begins fainting while in a seated position, Alejandro needs to immediately remove the needle, **secure** the patient, **treat** the patient, and then **document** the incident and ensure the patient's safety before she is released. The steps to follow are outlined below:

   ### Securing

   1. If the phlebotomy drawing chair has a bar that goes across the patient, the locked armrest can prevent a patient from falling.

   2. If the patient is beginning to faint and is not too heavy for the phlebotomist, the phlebotomist should support the patient and have the patient lower her head toward the floor and breathe deeply.

   3. If the patient is too heavy, the phlebotomist should support the patient with his or her own weight and call for help.

Treating

1. Use a cold compress on the forehead and the back of the neck.
2. Loosen tight clothing if possible.

Documenting/Ensuring Patient Safety

1. A supervisor should be informed and should talk to the patient or have the patient checked by an RN or physician.
2. The incident should be documented in the files.
3. The patient should not leave the laboratory for at least 15 minutes after he or she has recovered, and should refrain from driving for at least 30 minutes.

2. A blood pressure of 160/95 is abnormally high; potentially this patient's blood pressure is high because of hypertensive disease. After walking from the parking structure, this patient's blood pressure may be even higher because of exertion. The patient's blood pressure should be rechecked after resting and preferably before drawing the blood.

   A normal blood pressure is 120/80. The upper value is called the systolic pressure; this is the measurement of the blood pressure when the heart contracts. The lower value is called diastolic pressure; this is measured when the heart ventricles are relaxed and the atria are filling with blood.

3. Tubes required for collection:

   - T3 and T4
   - Liver panel, cholesterol
   - Triglycerides
   - One SST (serum separator tube)
   - Light green top, lithium heparin anticoagulant
   - One SST (serum separator tube)

   Tube requirements may vary because of methodology or instrumentation of various laboratories.

   No special transport conditions are necessary.

4. Proper tourniquet and vein selection techniques may help when obtaining blood from obese patients. Procedures that might help include:

   a. Tourniquet selection

      1. A regular tourniquet may be too short to function properly.
      2. Alternatives might be a blood pressure cuff, an extra-long Velcro closure strap, or an extra-long tourniquet.

   b. Vein selection

      1. If a patient has a double crease in the antecubital area, the median cubital vein may be palpable between creases.
      2. Sometimes turning the arm such that excess tissue redistributes to the lower part of the arm, thus exposing other veins, such as the cephalic vein, is helpful.
      3. Caution: Resist the temptation to probe because tissue, cell, and nerve damage can occur.

4. Do not forget the possibility of good veins in the hands.

5. Because of Mrs. L.M.'s weight and excess fatty tissue in her arms, it may be difficult to easily find a vein in the antecubital area. Alejandro evidently penetrated a nerve. The needle must be withdrawn immediately. He should then tell the patient that he or someone else will have to draw the blood at another time and that he will have a supervisor, RN, or physician examine the arm. An Incident Report must be completed and sent to administration. Nerve damage will usually show up days to weeks after an injury. Administration needs documentation of the occurrence in case it becomes a legal issue.

CASE 6
Repeat of a Newborn Screening Test

Baby M.S. is a 1-month-old infant and has been brought into the laboratory for a repeat PKU/newborn screening test. The laboratory receptionist has directed the baby and mother to a blood drawing room and has alerted a phlebotomist about a very young patient. Glenn is the phlebotomist who is available.

Key Words: heel stick • inherited metabolic disorders
• newborn screening test • PKU • restraining procedures for pediatrics

QUESTIONS

1. Would venipuncture or dermal puncture be an appropriate technique for obtaining a blood sample? Why?

2. Explain how each procedure (venipuncture, dermal puncture) is performed on an infant this size. What precautions need to be observed?

3. What would be the best procedure for restraining the child?

4. What is PKU or newborn screening?

DISCUSSION OF CASE STUDY

1. For a repeat newborn screening test, a capillary (dermal) puncture is performed with the blood collected on the same special filter paper provided for newborn screens. Capillary blood was collected for the original test, and capillary blood must be collected for the repeat screening test. Reference test values are based on levels of metabolites in capillary blood.

   • When performing capillary heel sticks (Fig. 1.5) for newborn screening, remember to fill each circle completely. Try not to overlap previously applied areas.

   • Air dry blood spots for 3 hours or until completely dry before processing the form. Before the specimen form can be sent to the newborn screening test site, a processing form must be filled out for each

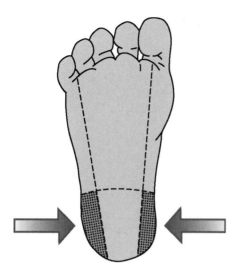

Figure 1.5. Heel stick. (Reprinted with permission from McCall RE, Tankersley CM. Phlebotomy Essentials. 3rd Ed. Philadelphia: Lippincott Williams & Wilkins, 2003.)

sample submitted. The processing form requires a newborn screening number, medical record number, and date of specimen.

- Fill in all information on the front of the form completely to avoid rejection of the specimen (Fig. 1.6).

If the repeat test is for a suspected abnormality detected from the initial newborn screening test, a syringe draw and venous blood may be

State of California—Health and Human Services Agency

CALIFORNIA NEWBORN SCREENING
TEST REQUEST FORM (TRF)

Department of Health Services

Apply barcode from filter paper card here.

PLEASE PRINT USING ALL CAPITAL LETTERS

NEWBORN
LAST NAME | FIRST | MULTIPLE A, B, C ...
ADDRESS: NUMBER | STREET | APARTMENT
CITY | STATE | ZIP CODE

MALE | FEMALE | BIRTH WEIGHT | GMS

(FOR AREA SCREENING LABORATORY USE ONLY)

NEWBORN'S BIRTH DATE:
MONTH | DAY | YEAR | HOUR

DATE SPECIMEN COLLECTED:
MONTH | DAY | YEAR | HOUR

MOTHER
MOTHER'S LAST NAME | FIRST | M. I.
MOTHER'S MAIDEN NAME | SOCIAL SECURITY NUMBER
AREA CODE | PHONE | MOTHER'S BIRTH DATE: MONTH | DAY | YEAR

INITIALS OF COLLECTOR:

TYPE OF SPECIMEN:
HEELSTICK
OTHER (Specify):

IF COLLECTED AT < 12 HRS OF AGE, REASON:
TO BE TRANSFUSED
OTHER (Specify):

NEWBORN'S PHYSICIAN
LAST NAME | FIRST
ADDRESS: NUMBER | STREET | SUITE
CITY | STATE | ZIP CODE
AREA CODE | PHONE | X | LICENSE NUMBER

RBC TRANSFUSION BEFORE COLLECTION:
NO | YES
If YES, date/time last transfusion completed:
MONTH | DAY | YEAR | HOUR

RACE/ETHNICITY: FILL ALL THAT APPLY
WHITE | KOREAN | FILIPINO | SAMOAN
HISPANIC | VIETNAMESE | MIDDLE EASTERN | NATIVE AMERICAN
BLACK | CAMBODIAN | ASIAN-EAST INDIAN | OTHER (Specify):
CHINESE | LAOTIAN (LAOS) | HAWAIIAN
JAPANESE | OTHER S.E. ASIAN | GUAMANIAN

REASON FOR TEST (Fill only ONE box.):
INITIAL SPECIMEN
REPEAT OF INADEQUATE INITIAL SPECIMEN
REPEAT OF EARLY (<12 HRS) INITIAL SPECIMEN
OTHER REPEAT (Specify):

PRIMARY LANGUAGE (Fill only ONE box.):
ENGLISH | SPANISH | OTHER (Specify):

IF PATIENT HAS MEDI-CAL, WRITE MEDI-CAL #, BIC OR PE# HERE:

FACILITY DRAWING SPECIMEN: | HOSPITAL CODE

ALL FEEDINGS SINCE BIRTH (Fill only ONE box.):
BREAST ONLY | TPN/HYPERAL
FORMULA ONLY | OTHER (Specify):
BREAST & FORMULA

NURSERY TYPE:
NICU | REGULAR NURSERY | OTHER (Specify):

MEDICAL RECORD #:

White copy—must accompany specimen. Goldenrod copy—file in newborn's chart.

PLEASE SEE PRIVACY NOTIFICATION ON REVERSE

DHS 4409 (3/05) To reorder, request form NBS-TRF from the Genetic Disease Branch, Newborn Screening Section (510) 412-3950. NBS-I (AA)

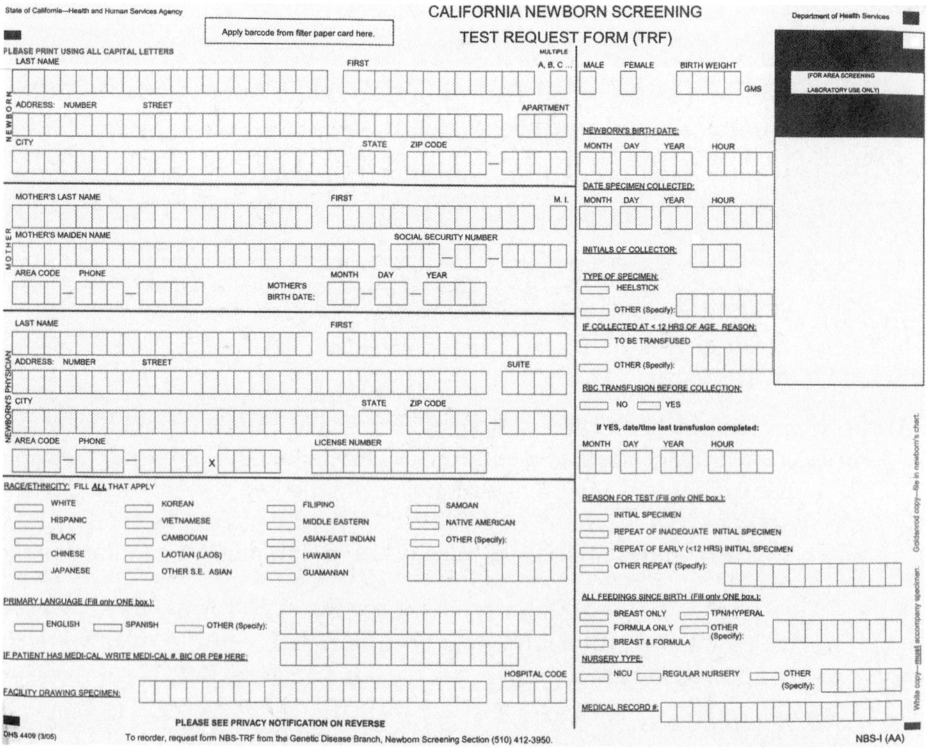

Figure 1.6. Newborn Screening Test Request Form and Specimen Collection Card.

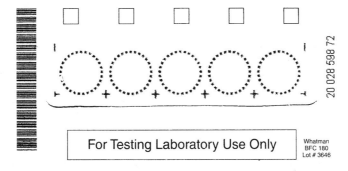

For Testing Laboratory Use Only

Whatman
BFC 180
Lot # 3646

20 028 598 72

Completed Test Request Form (TRF) must accompany specimen.

Apply Labels to TRF

20 028 598 72

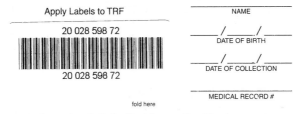

20 028 598 72

fold here

NAME
_____

_____ / _____ / _____
DATE OF BIRTH

_____ / _____ / _____
DATE OF COLLECTION

_____
MEDICAL RECORD #

Instructions for Collecting Adequate Blood Specimens

Do not use capillary tubes for collection of blood spot specimen. **Do not** collect blood from intravenous/intra-arterial lines, antecubital space or dorsal hand veins. **Do not** handle blood collection area of specimen collection prior to, during, or following sampling.

1. Position infant's foot to increase blood flow. Warming of heel is optional.
2. Clean skin with alcohol and either air-dry or wipe dry with sterile gauze.
3. Puncture heel with sterile disposable lancet, using a firm, quick stab. If using an automated lancet device, place it firmly against the heel prior to device activation.
4. Allow a large drop of blood to accumulate; wipe away with sterile gauze.
5. Allow a second large drop of blood to accumulate. Apply gentle pressure to heel and ease intermittently so blood flows freely.
6. Apply the blood drop to one side of the specimen collection paper until the circle is filled COMPLETELY when viewed from both sides. Do not press collection paper against puncture site. Allow blood to fill circle by natural flow. **Do not apply blood to both sides of the paper.**
7. Fill the first circle completely before moving on to the next circle. Repeat procedure for each circle.
8. Allow blood spots to air-dry at room temperature for at least three hours. Keep away from direct light (sun or lamp) and heat.
9. Do not close specimen collection form or place in plastic bag while blood spots are still wet. Do not allow wet specimens to come in contact with each other.

fold here

California
Newborn
Screening

Specimen
Collection
Card

INSTRUCTIONS FOR COLLECTING ADEQUATE BLOOD SPECIMENS

Puncture site is indicated by shaded areas on heel. Do not collect from side or back of foot.

NO

RIGHT	Acceptable	WRONG	Unacceptable
	Circle filled and evenly saturated		Layering
			Insufficient, multiple applications
			Serum rings present

Figure 1.6.   (*Continued*)

recommended for the confirmation tests. Glenn needs to indicate the source of blood when sending the screening test back.

2. Capillary heel puncture: Refer to a phlebotomy manual for correct heel puncture techniques. Remember to use a heel warmer and the correct lancet size for the infant's weight. To ensure a good flow of blood for acceptable specimen submission, massage the area for heel puncture, and use the squeeze-and-release collection method. By releasing pressure on the heel, blood flows into the capillaries and hemolysis and excess tissue fluid is avoided.

   If other blood tests are ordered, a venipuncture may also be necessary. Glenn should use a dorsal hand vein and a 23-gauge butterfly, 3-mL syringe. No tourniquet or Band-Aid should be used. The infant could pull off the Band-Aid and place it in his or her mouth. Refer to a phlebotomy manual for complete procedures.

3. What would be the best procedure for restraining the child?

   • Wrapping the infant in a receiving blanket is a good restraining method.
   • Have the parent or an assistant restrain the arms and free leg of the infant.

4. Newborn screening tests are used to detect inherited metabolic disorders. A metabolic disorder can cause severe brain damage if not detected and treatment is not started early. US law mandates screening on all newborns for hypothyroidism and phenylketonuria (PKU). Other states require screening for other metabolic disorders, sickle cell, etc.

Quiz

MULTIPLE CHOICE:

1. Patient A.K. has a broken arm and a cast on the left arm. The right arm has an IV drip running. Where is the optimal site for drawing blood?
   a. dorsal right foot
   b. left hand
   c. right hand below the IV
   d. right dorsal hand below the IV
   e. c and d

2. Which statement is *not* true of type I diabetes?
   a. more common in childhood
   b. insulin deficiency occurs
   c. insulin resistance occurs
   d. blood glucose becomes elevated
   e. Diabetes is a metabolic, endocrine disorder.

3. Mrs. S.J. had a mastectomy 3 years ago on her left side. Where is the optimal site for drawing blood?
   a. vein in the left antecubital area
   b. left hand vein
   c. vein in the right antecubital area
   d. right hand vein
   e. c and d

4. With a mastectomy, cancerous breast tissue and _____ are removed.
   a. adjacent axillary lymph nodes
   b. cervical lymph nodes
   c. atrial lymph nodes
   d. medial sternal lymph nodes
   e. inguinal lymph nodes

5. The major blood vessel entering the right atrium of the heart is the _____.
   a. subclavian vein
   b. pulmonary vein
   c. pulmonary artery
   d. superior vena cava
   e. jugular vein

6. Tissue or a graft donated from another person is called _____.
   a. autologous
   b. allogeneic
   c. xenogeneic
   d. syngeneic
   e. homologous

7. The minimum amount of blood needed for a CBC is _____.
   a. 8 mL
   b. 5 mL
   c. 1 mL
   d. 0.5 mL
   e. 0.25 mL

8. The minimum amount of blood needed for electrolytes is _____.
   a. 10 mL
   b. 8 mL
   c. 5 mL
   d. 2 mL
   e. 1 mL

9. Which of the following is incorrect for obtaining a blood sample from a vascular access device (VAD)?

   a. The phlebotomist may draw the blood sample.

   b. The first 5 mL of blood drawn from a VAD should be discarded.

   c. The VAD needs to be flushed with saline or heparin.

   d. Sterile technique should be used in accessing the device.

   e. The phlebotomist needs to indicate that the blood sample was drawn from a VAD.

10. The preferred site for obtaining blood for a CBC from a 2-year-old child is____.

   a. finger stick

   b. heel stick

   c. venipuncture antecubital area

   d. venipuncture dorsal hand

   e. dermal puncture of big toe

11. The optimal needle size for a venipuncture from a 2-year-old child is _____.

   a. 20 gauge

   b. 21 gauge

   c. 23 gauge

   d. 25 gauge

12. Which blood tests usually require the patient to be fasting at the time the blood sample is drawn?

   a. thyroid

   b. cholesterol

   c. triglycerides

   d. a and b

   e. b and c

13. Conditions that may lead to fainting include _____.

   a. low blood sugar

   b. high blood pressure

   c. rapid heart beat rate

   d. a and b

   e. a, b, and c

14. The top number on a blood pressure reading is called _____ and represents the blood pressure when the heart is _____.

   a. diastolic . . . contracting

   b. diastolic . . . at rest

   c. systolic . . . contracting

   d. systolic . . . at rest

15. Which blood test requires that the blood sample be transported in an ice slurry?
    a. T3 and T4
    b. ammonia
    c. triglycerides
    d. a and b
    e. b and c

16. Screening tests for metabolic diseases in newborn infants require ____ blood obtained from ____.
    a. venous . . . venipuncture
    b. capillary . . . a heel stick
    c. arterial . . . a heel stick
    d. venous . . . a heel stick
    e. arterial . . . a scalp vein

MATCHING
Answers may be used more than once or not at all.

17. Stat		a.	mathematical reference
18. glucometer		b.	yellow coloring to the skin
19. edema		c.	point-of-care instrument
20. jaundice		d.	results needed as rapidly as possible
		e.	increased tissue fluids

21. CVC		a.	metabolic disease
22. PKU		b.	breakaway cancer cells
23. PICC		c.	vascular access device
24. metastatic		d.	donor tissue
25. allogeneic		e.	cancer test

MATCH CORRECT TUBES TO TEST

26. lead		a.	red
27. cholesterol		b.	lavender
28. potassium		c.	green
		d.	royal blue
		e.	a and c

29. liver panel   a. green tube

30. CBC   b. red, gold, or green

31. ESR   c. lavender

                                          d. black

                                          e. c and d

SHORT ESSAY

32. What is a point-of-care instrument? Include in your description an example of a POC and when it is appropriate to use a POC instrument.

33. What is a mastectomy? Why does the phlebotomist need to be aware of on which side a mastectomy has occurred?

34. Describe at least three techniques that can help make drawing blood from a child less stressful.

35. Describe three techniques for restraining small children who need to have blood drawn.

36. Describe the optimum technique for obtaining a blood sample from the antecubital area of a very overweight person. Name an alternative site.

37. Outline the subsequent steps to be taken if a patient experiences a sharp pain at the site of venipuncture in addition to the minimal pain when the needle enters the skin.

38. Describe the technique for obtaining a blood sample for a newborn metabolic screening test.

39. Describe at least two techniques for restraining an infant while obtaining a blood sample by heel puncture.

40. Describe the optimum procedure for obtaining a blood sample from an infant by venipuncture.

CHAPTER 2

Coagulation

CASE 7
Inadequate Tube Fill

Rosa is the phlebotomist in charge of collecting a CBC and prothrombin time (PT) from Mrs. R.S. Rosa follows correct procedure and is able to enter the vein with a Vacutainer with no problem. However, as she is collecting the blood for the PT, a brief spurt of blood enters the tube and then she hears a hissing sound. The blood stops flowing. She repositions the needle, but is not able to establish blood flow.

Key Words: anticoagulant-to-blood ratio • discard tube for coagulation studies • loss of vacuum • order of draw • prothrombin time • sodium citrate • tissue fluid fibrin • Vacutainer tubes

QUESTIONS

1. What tubes are necessary for the CBC and PT?

2. Is there a particular order that should be followed for drawing these blood samples?

3. Why did the blood flow stop in the PT tube? Is the blood sample useful for testing?

4. What can Rosa do to correct the problem?

DISCUSSION OF CASE STUDY

1. Tubes necessary for the PT and CBC are:

   • One blue-top tube completely filled for the PT
   • One lavender-top tube for the CBC

2. Using a Vacutainer, the order of draw should be first the blue-top tube and then the lavender-top tube. The PT tube contains sodium citrate as the anticoagulant. Sodium citrate binds calcium. Calcium in the blood is essential for formation of fibrin (Fig. 2.1).

   Fibrin is the protein that forms a mesh or net that stops blood flow from a wound site. Sodium citrate works as an anticoagulant by

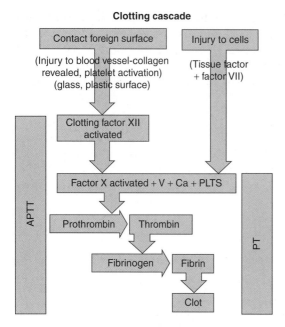

Clotting cascade

Figure 2.1. Clotting Cascade.

binding to the calcium, and thereby calcium is unavailable for clotting.

The lavender-top tube also contains an anticoagulant—EDTA (ethylene diamine tetra-acetic acid). The lavender-top tube is drawn last to ensure that this anticoagulant does not contaminate the tube for the PT test.

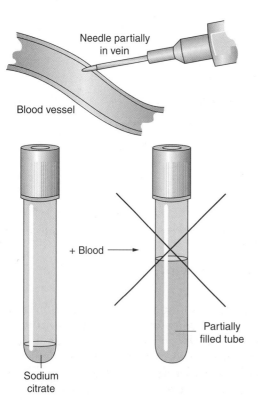

Figure 2.2. Inadequate Tube Fill.

3. The blood stopped flowing because the needle was pulled partially out of the vein, allowing the vacuum to escape from the blue-top tube. With loss of vacuum, no further blood is drawn into the tube. A very precise concentration of sodium citrate to blood must be present in the tube for accurate test results. This blue-top tube was not filled completely, and thus this tube is unusable (Fig. 2.2).

4. When the needle re-entered the vein, the blue-top tube had lost its vacuum, thus there was no vacuum to pull blood from the vein. If the blue-top tube were replaced with a new tube, with the vacuum intact, the blood draw could continue. However, if blood still does not flow into the new tube, Rosa will need to withdraw the Vacutainer from the vein and draw from the other arm.

CASE 8
Patient on "Blood Thinner"

Mr. E.S. is an elderly gentleman who experienced a heart attack 2 months ago. Fortunately it was a fairly mild attack, and he has walked into the blood drawing center to have blood drawn for a liver panel and PT. He mentions to Eduardo, the phlebotomist, that he is taking a "blood thinner."

Key Words: arteriosclerosis • blood thinner • Coumadin • order of draw • warfarin

QUESTIONS

1. What tubes are necessary for these tests?
2. Is there a particular order that is necessary for collection of the tests?
3. What type of "blood thinner" is he most likely taking?
4. What special precautions should the phlebotomist take?

DISCUSSION OF CASE STUDY

1. The liver panel requires a red-top tube, although some laboratories may be able to perform the liver panel tests on heparinized plasma in a green-top tube. The PT requires a blue-top tube.

2. Using a Vacutainer and plastic tubes, the order of draw would be blue, red, and green.

3. The patient is probably taking Coumadin. Coumadin is the brand name for sodium warfarin. Warfarin is an anticoagulant that directly inhibits coagulation factor production. One of the most common causes of a heart attack is arteriosclerosis (hardening of the arteries). Unfortunately, the most vulnerable blood vessels for developing arteriosclerosis are blood vessels that supply the heart muscle and brain with O_2 and

nutrients. The walls of these blood vessels become hardened, and the interior space becomes clogged with cholesterol plaques. Should platelets adhere to these uneven surfaces and activate the clotting factors, a clot occurs. The blood vessel becomes completely blocked, and the patient suffers heart attack or stroke.

Once having suffered a heart attack or stroke, the patient is given heparin to prevent further clots and to allow time for the present clot to dissolve. Heparin must be given by injection or intravenously. To release the patient and send him or her home, it is more convenient to switch the medication to an oral anticoagulant such as Coumadin. To ensure that the Coumadin is suppressing clotting activity (acting as a blood thinner), the PT test must be performed. To ensure that the patient is not taking too little or too much and the dosage is correct, the prothrombin test must be accurate. Accuracy is dependent on venipuncture technique and quality of the blood sample.

4. Special precautions that the phlebotomist needs to take include applying pressure for a longer period of time after withdrawing the needle. Because Mr. E.S. is taking medication that suppresses clotting, he will have a tendency to bleed more easily. Pressure should be applied to the venipuncture site for 2 to 5 minutes. Eduardo should check the site to make sure clotting has occurred and there is no further bleeding.

CASE 9
Prothrombin Time

Mr. S.K. is an 80-year-old black man who comes to the laboratory to have his prothrombin time (PT) checked. When Christine, the phlebotomist, drew the blood, she drew a red-top tube and two blue-top tubes. She drew two blue-top tubes because the first blue-top tube stopped filling at one quarter of the tube. She noticed that the second tube was not quite full enough either, so she placed some blood from the first blue-top tube into the second blue-top tube to fill the tube completely. The specimens remained in the outpatient blood-drawing center for 5 hours before being taken along with other tubes to the Hematology Department of the laboratory. The results were longer than expected. Mr. S.K. had commented to Christine that he was taking a "blood thinner" and had been following instructions given by the physician very carefully.

Key Words: anticoagulant • coagulation tube ratio • Coumadin • platelet plug • sodium citrate • specimen integrity

QUESTIONS

1. Do you think the results are accurate?

2. What anticoagulant is in a blue-top tube? How does it work?

3. If the results are incorrect, what might have caused the incorrect results?

4. Why did the phlebotomist draw a red-top tube before drawing the blue-top tube?

5. Should any special precautions be taken with the patient?

6. What type of "blood thinner" is he most likely taking?

DISCUSSION OF CASE STUDY

1. The results of the PT are definitely <u>not</u> accurate.

2. The anticoagulant in the blue-top tube is sodium citrate. The sodium citrate combines with calcium in the blood to form an insoluble calcium salt. This removes calcium from the blood sample. To have optimum activity of platelets and clotting factors, calcium is necessary. If calcium is unavailable, clotting cannot occur. Prothrombin is one of the clotting factors inhibited by a "blood thinner." When a prothrombin test is performed, plasma is separated, additional calcium is added, and then the time it takes for the specimen to clot is measured.

3. Test results will definitely be inaccurate because the processing of the tubes was delayed for 5 hours. Clotting factors are fragile proteins that do not remain active at room temperature for very long. After 4 hours, the integrity of the specimen is questionable. Each laboratory must determine how many hours they will allow before a specimen is considered unacceptable.

In addition, adding blood from another specimen tube has compromised the ratio of anticoagulant to blood. By mixing the blood sample of a different tube, the ratio of blood to anticoagulant is totally "off." The correct ratio for coagulation tubes is 9 parts blood to 1 part anticoagulant. A phlebotomist should NEVER transfer blood from one tube to another.

4. A glass red-top tube or plastic BD light red (contains no clot activator) or blue or black discard tube must be used before drawing a blue-top tube to prevent tissue fluid contamination. Some laboratories believe that the amount of tissue fluid contamination is not enough to interfere with prothrombin and partial thromboplastin times. Each laboratory should perform its own studies to determine whether a predraw tube is necessary.

The use of a predraw discard tube is being presented here to introduce the concept of coagulation activation by tissue contamination factors.

5. When drawing blood from a patient who is on anticoagulant therapy, extra precautions should be taken to confirm that the patient has stopped bleeding. Maintain pressure on the venipuncture site for 2 to 5 minutes. Christine needs to be aware that patients on anticoagulant therapy may not form an initial good platelet plug. If this happens, the patient may move his or her arm and start bleeding again. Confirm that the platelet plug has formed well enough to prevent further bleeding.

6. The patient is probably taking Coumadin. Coumadin is the brand name for the active ingredient warfarin. Warfarin is an anticoagulant that inhibits vitamin K-dependent coagulation factors (Fig. 2.3).

Vitamin K - dependent clotting factors

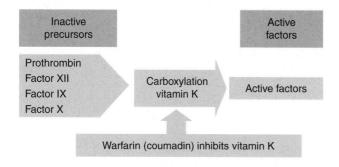

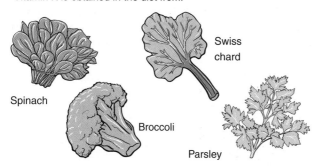

Vitamin K is obtained in the diet from:

Spinach

Swiss chard

Broccoli

Parsley

A good reason to eat your greens!

Figure 2.3. Vitamin K-dependent Clotting Factor.

CASE 10
Karyotyping

Mrs. R.P. is a 58-year-old white woman who needs blood drawn for karyotyping. Her previous complete blood count (CBC) indicated a white blood cell (WBC) count of 350,000 cells/mm³. She is very distraught and asks you to tell her what this number means.

Key Words: chromosomes • heparin • HIPAA • karyotype • lithium • mitosis • sodium heparin

QUESTIONS

1. What is karyotyping?

2. What anticoagulant is needed?

3. What do you tell the patient? What is HIPAA?

DISCUSSION OF CASE STUDY

1. Karyotyping is a special procedure that involves growing blood cells in tissue culture. White blood cells are induced to undergo mitosis, and then at metaphase the mitotic process is stopped. When a cell begins mitosis, it first duplicates its DNA and then condenses and coils the DNA

strands into individual chromosomes. At metaphase the duplicated chromosomes are aligned at the center of the cell and are ready to migrate to the opposite ends to form two new cells. To prepare a karyotype, a picture is taken of the duplicate chromosomes and the chromosomes are then arranged according to size. A normal karyotype will show an array of 23 pairs of chromosomes, including two sex chromosomes. A patient's karyotype is then compared for normal size, shape, and number. Down syndrome is also called trisomy 21 because in a Down syndrome patient there are three #21 chromosomes instead of only two. Cancer cells will also show abnormal karyotypes (Fig. 2.4 and Fig. 2.5).

Blood specimens and bone marrow specimens are drawn to analyze for hematological disorders that are identified by specific chromosome abnormalities.

2. Sodium heparin is the anticoagulant necessary for a karyotype. The blood cells must be grown in cell culture to perform a karyotype. Sodium heparin best preserves the cells in a living (viable) condition.

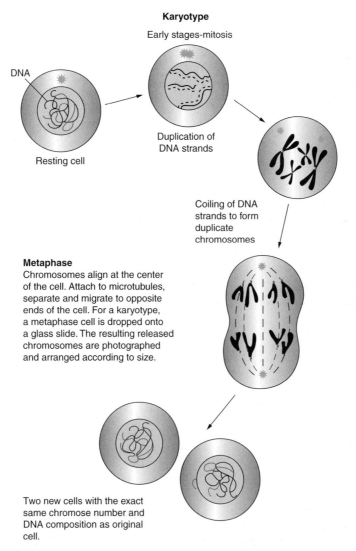

Figure 2.4. Flow Chart of Mitosis, Metaphase Chromosomes.

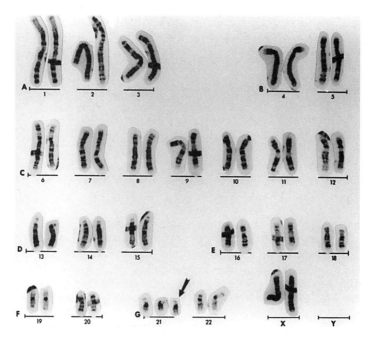

Figure 2.5. A Trisomy 21 Karyotype. (Reprinted with permission from Dr. Kathleen Rao, Department of Pediatrics, University of North Carolina.)

Why not use lithium heparin?

Lithium is toxic to blood cells, thus care must be taken to use green-top tubes with sodium heparin instead of lithium heparin.

Transport at room temperature immediately. Remember, you are working with live cells. Most specimens must be received at the testing laboratory within 48 hours. Clinical and patient history must be included.

3. When a patient or family member asks for an explanation of their tests, you should refer them to their physician for an explanation. In addition, just because a family member is in the room does not mean that the patient wants that person to know about his medical problems. According to HIPAA, a patient must agree before information can be released about his or her condition. HIPAA, the Health Insurance Portability and Accountability Act, is a law enacted by the US Congress to protect the confidentiality of electronic transfer of patients' medical records. It has grown to encompass patient confidentiality throughout the hospital, doctors' offices, clinics, etc.

CASE 11
Complications in a Postpartum Patient

Mrs. C.A. is a 28-year-old white woman who was recently transferred from the labor and delivery department. A CBC, PT, PTT, and blood glucose were ordered for her. The patient was not very responsive, and her skin was cold and clammy. Anticipating further orders, the phlebotomist drew an additional red-top tube and proceeded to draw blood for the rest of the patients on her list. While separating tubes in the laboratory, the phlebotomist noticed that the blood from Mrs. C.A. in the red-top tube had not clotted.

Key Words: D-dimers • DIC • FDPs • fibrinogen • platelets • postpartum

QUESTIONS

1. What are possible causes for the blood not clotting in the red-top tube?

2. Why is the patient cold and clammy?

3. What should the phlebotomist do?

DISCUSSION OF CASE STUDY

1. Mrs. C.A. was recently transferred from labor and delivery. She may have experienced complications during delivery, and the child may not have survived. Having delivered the child, Mrs. C.A. is now considered postpartum.

It seems that the patient's blood is *not* clotting. Ample time for clot formation has occurred since Mrs. C.A.'s blood was drawn. Reasons for lack of blood clotting could be decreased platelets, decreased fibrinogen, and other clotting factors. A complication that can occur in obstetric patients is a condition called DIC (disseminated intravascular coagulation). Disseminated refers to the widespread dissemination throughout the blood vessels (intravascular) of tiny microclots. Fibrin is being formed and becomes entangled with RBCs and platelets. These tiny clots consume platelets and clotting factors circulating in the blood. The body attempts to break down these clots, and fibrin degradation products (FDPs) are released. FDPs inhibit clotting. At the same time that the patient is forming clots, she is at risk for bleeding problems because of inhibition and consumption of platelets and clotting factors. The decrease in platelets and clotting factors compromises the patient's ability to control her bleeding. Death can occur if the DIC is not stopped (Fig. 2.6).

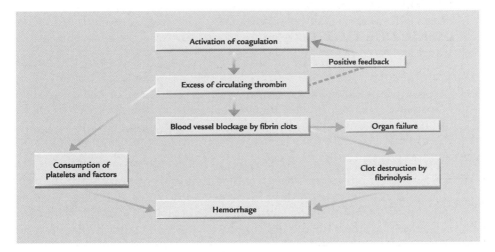

Figure 2.6.   DIC Diagram. (Reprinted with permission from Anatomical Chart Co.)

2. The patient is cold and clammy and is not very responsive because she is probably unconscious and in shock.

3. The phlebotomist should inform the laboratory hematologist about the nonclotted specimen. The nurse in charge of this patient should also be notified of the patient's condition. Immediate action needs to be taken. Mrs. C.A.'s physician needs to be informed. Laboratory tests can be ordered to confirm that Mrs. C.A. has DIC. Useful tests include platelet count, RBC morphology, fibrinogen level, D-dimer assays, and DIC panel for fibrin degradation products.

CASE 12
Unstoppable Nose Bleed

T.J. is a 5-year-old boy whose mother is Filipino and does not understand English very well. T.J. was admitted in the emergency room with a nosebleed that has been unstoppable for the past 2 hours. The doctor has ordered a CBC with platelet count and PT and PTT. As the phlebotomist, you also notice that the child has numerous bruises on the arms and face.

Key Words: bleeding disorders • child abuse • hemophilia • patient identification

QUESTIONS

1. How do you establish identification and explain what you need to do?

2. Where is the best site for obtaining a blood sample? Explain your procedure.

3. What tubes do you need? Are there any special precautions that you should follow? Are there any legal precautions that you should take?

DISCUSSION OF CASE STUDY

1. You will need an interpreter to confirm identification of the patient and to explain the procedure. The mother does not understand English well enough to understand your explanation of the procedure. She needs to understand to give consent to draw blood from her child, and you may need her cooperation in holding the child. Even if the child speaks English, he is too traumatized and too young to serve as an interpreter.

2. A 5-year-old child's veins are developed enough to draw from the antecubital fossa. Do not tie the tourniquet too tightly. Excessive pressure may cause more bruising. Even though bruising from the tourniquet might occur, blood for the clotting tests (PT, PTT) can only be obtained from a venipuncture.

3. You should draw a blue-top tube for PT and PTT and a lavender-top tube for CBC.

4. The child's bruises may be caused by a bleeding disorder, such as hemophilia, thrombocytopenia (decreased platelets), or possibly by child abuse. A complication of viral pneumonia causes loss of platelets. If the number of platelets in the blood circulation becomes too low, bruising can occur. The physician and nursing staff will determine if the bruising is from a clinical condition or from abuse. If abuse is suspected, the necessary authorities must be alerted.

CASE 13
Petechiae

Ms. T.M. is a 25-year-old white woman who needs a bleeding time. She has numerous bruises and petechiae on her arms.

Key Words: aspirin ingestion • autoimmune disease • bleeding time • petechiae • platelet plug • primary hemostasis • spleen

QUESTIONS

1. What are petechiae?

2. How is a bleeding time performed? What equipment is necessary? Explain the procedure.

3. How is aspirin related?

DISCUSSION OF CASE STUDY

1. Petechiae are tiny bruises or red spots (speckles) that appear on the skin or mucous membranes (Fig. 2.7). These speckles may occur spontaneously or after minor trauma. The most common cause for formation of petechiae is decreased platelets (thrombocytopenia). So, what causes the platelets to become decreased? In the case of Ms. T.M., she may have developed antibodies to her own platelets. This is referred to as an autoimmune disease. The antibodies bind to the platelets, and the platelets are then removed from the circulation by the spleen. The spleen is a small organ located above the left kidney that has a large blood supply. The spleen's normal function is to remove old RBCs. However, any particles coated with antibodies will also be removed. The number of platelets in the circulation can be determined by performing a platelet count.

2. Petechiae and bruising may occur because of a decreased number of platelets or inadequate function of the platelets. A bleeding time is a screening test for measuring the interaction of platelets with the blood vessel wall, which leads to platelet plug formation and stoppage of bleeding. The bleeding time is prolonged when the platelet level is low or they cannot adhere to the wounded vessel wall. Normal platelet plug formation occurs in a series of steps referred to as primary hemostasis.

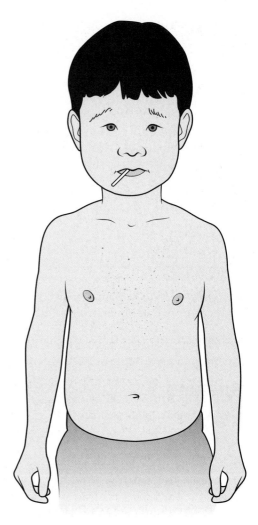

Figure 2.7. Small Boy with Petechiae.
(LifeART image copyright © (2006)
Lippincott Williams & Wilkins. All rights
reserved.)

The steps for primary hemostasis are:

a. Vasoconstriction to decrease the flow of blood to the injured area
b. Platelet adhesion to the injured area
c. Platelet aggregation—clumping of platelets, adherence to each other
d. Platelet plug formation (Fig. 2.8)

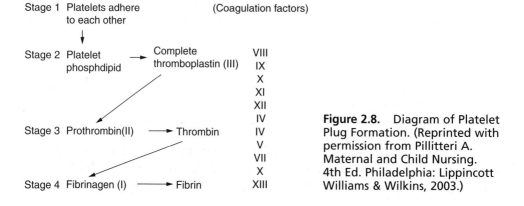

Figure 2.8. Diagram of Platelet
Plug Formation. (Reprinted with
permission from Pillitteri A.
Maternal and Child Nursing.
4th Ed. Philadelphia: Lippincott
Williams & Wilkins, 2003.)

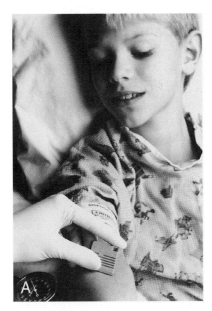
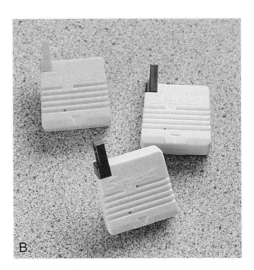

Figure 2.9. Simplate Device. (Reprinted with permission from McCall RE, Tankersley CM. Phlebotomy Essentials. 3rd Ed. Philadelphia: Lippincott Williams & Wilkins, 2003.)

Note: Platelet plug formation is sufficient for injuries such as needle puncture. Larger injuries require secondary hemostasis, which is the formation of a larger clot consisting of RBCs, platelets, and fibrin.

A common bleeding time test is called the IVY bleeding time, and a Simplate II incision device is used (Fig. 2.9).

Procedure: A blood pressure cuff is applied to the arm and inflated to 40 mm Hg. This is maintained throughout the test. An incision on the forearm is performed using the Simplate device. Seepage of blood from the incision is blotted with filter paper every 30 seconds. Be careful to not dislodge the forming clot when blotting the excess blood. Bleeding should cease within 5 to 7 minutes. Prolonged times can be from more than 7 minutes to over 20 minutes.

Any surgical procedure should be delayed or cancelled if a bleeding time is prolonged until the cause of the prolonged bleeding time is determined.

3. Aspirin can affect the ability of the platelets to adhere to each other and the vessel wall. Thus, a defective platelet plug is formed that will extend the bleeding time. A patient should refrain from taking aspirin for at least 10 days before surgery. The effect of aspirin exists for the life span of the platelet. The life span of a platelet is less than 10 days. Therefore, when surgery does occur, a new population of platelets, not exposed to aspirin, will exist.

CASE 14
Low Fibrinogen

An 18-year-old woman has just delivered a baby and is having problems with bleeding. The physician orders CBC, CHEM7, PT, PTT, fibrinogen, and FDP (fibrin degradation products). The phlebotomist draws the patient with a syringe that fills up very slowly. She fills the Vacutainer tubes in the following order: gold, green, blue, and lavender tops. The results indicate a normal CBC except low platelets; normal PT, PTT, and FDP; but low fibrinogen. The doctor wants the patient's blood samples redrawn. The patient's blood was redrawn with a butterfly attached to a Vacutainer holder. The second results were all normal.

Key Words: anticoagulant • chemistry • disseminated intravascular coagulation (DIC) • fibrinogen • hematology • partial thromboplastin time • prothrombin time

QUESTIONS

1. Why would the physician want the specimen(s) redrawn?

2. Did the phlebotomist draw everything properly?

3. What tube was drawn for each test, and what was the anticoagulant for each tube? Should any test require special handling? What departments performed the tests?

4. What diagnosis was the physician trying to rule out?

DISCUSSION OF CASE STUDY

1. The phlebotomist drew the patient's specimens with a syringe that filled very slowly. The physician suspects a clotted specimen because of the results of low platelets and low fibrinogen. A clot could have adhered to the side of one of the tubes and escaped detection. Numerous microclots might occur without detection as well. Any clot formation will use up platelets and fibrinogen. Because the redraw specimen results were normal, the original specimen must have been clotted.

2. The phlebotomist did not observe the correct order of draw. The correct order of draw is: discard tube, blue-top, gold-top, green-top, and lavender-top tubes.

3. Blue-top tubes are for coagulation studies in the hematology department.
    Tests such as PT, PTT, fibrinogen, and FDPs are performed. The specimen tube must be filled completely and mixed gently 10 to 15 times. The anticoagulant is sodium citrate, which binds with calcium to prevent clotting.
    Green-top tubes are for chemistry studies in the chemistry department. Common tests are chemistry panels, cardiac enzymes, liver enzymes, etc. Specimen tubes should be mixed gently 10 to 15 times. The anticoagulant is lithium heparin, which inactivates thrombin to prevent clotting.
    Lavender-top tubes are for hematology studies. Common tests are CBC, platelet counts, WBC differential, reticulocyte count, etc. Specimen tubes should be mixed gently 10 to 15 times. The anticoagulant is EDTA, which binds with calcium to prevent clotting.

4. DIC will use up fibrinogen as it forms clots and breaks up clots into fibrin degradation products, thus needing more fibrinogen to form more clots.

CASE 15
Simplate Bleeding Time

An arthritic 50-year-old woman is undergoing knee surgery. While in the surgery holding area, the phlebotomist performs a Simplate bleeding time on the patient. The result is abnormal. The patient's CBC performed earlier in the week for preoperative screening was normal, including the platelets. The physician asks for the bleeding time to be repeated. The results are still abnormal.

Key Words: anti-inflammatory agents • platelet dysfunction • platelet function assays • Simplate bleeding time

QUESTIONS

1. What would cause an abnormal bleeding time?
2. Could a phlebotomist's technique cause an abnormal result?
3. Who is qualified to perform a bleeding time?
4. What is the Simplate bleeding time measuring?
5. What test could the physician order to obtain the same information?

DISCUSSION OF CASE STUDY

1. Causes of an abnormal bleeding time include:
   a. Anti-inflammatory agents such as aspirin
      Antimicrobial agents in high doses
      Penicillin (-cillin drugs such as ampicillin)
      Cephalosporins
   b. Low platelets or an anemic patient
   c. Platelet dysfunctions
2. Bleeding time results are *very* dependent on technique.
   If the Simplate device is pressed down on the forearm with too much pressure, a larger, deeper cut will be made, which will increase the bleeding time. If the pressure is not enough, a decreased bleeding time will occur. If the filter paper dislodges the forming platelet plug, the time will be extended.
3. In a few states, only the clinical laboratory scientist (CLS) or medical technologist (MT) is allowed to perform a bleeding time. In the majority

of states, a clinical laboratory technician (CLT) or phlebotomist performs the bleeding times.

4. The Simplate bleeding time is a screening test to measure the interaction of the platelets to the damaged blood vessel walls, platelet adhesiveness, and platelet plug formation.

5. A platelet function assay is more accurate than the bleeding time. It is a precise measurement of the platelets' ability to clot. The test takes approximately 1 hour to perform, but does eliminate the variation in techniques associated with the bleeding time.

Quiz

MULTIPLE CHOICE

1. What is the proper order of draw? Note: All tubes are plastic with clot activator.
   a. blue, lavender, and green
   b. yellow (SPS), green, lavender, and blue
   c. blue, green, and lavender
   d. yellow (SPS), blue, green, and lavender

2. When drawing a blue-top tube, which of the following is correct?
   a. Fill tube to line or vacuum draw.
   b. A ratio of 4.5 mL whole blood to 0.5 mL sodium citrate anticoagulant is required in each tube.
   c. A ratio of 1.0 mL sodium citrate to 9.0 mL whole blood is required in each tube.
   d. a and b are correct
   e. a, b, and c are correct

3. Primary hemostasis involves the following steps in the following order.
   a. platelet aggregation, vasoconstriction, platelet adhesion, and platelet plug formation
   b. vasoconstriction, platelet aggregation, platelet adhesion, and platelet plug formation
   c. platelet aggregation, platelet adhesion, vasoconstriction, and platelet plug formation
   d. vasoconstriction, plate adhesion, platelet aggregation, and platelet plug formation

4. When blood is circulating in the body, the liquid that carries the cells is:
   a. serum
   b. saline
   c. plasma
   d. water

MATCHING
Refer to diagram labeled a, b, or c.

5. Where would you find RBCs?

6. Where would you find platelets?

7. Where would you find clotting factors?

8. Where would you find WBCs?

9. Where would you find fibrinogen?

10. Where would you find plasma?

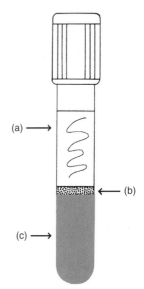

SELECT THE CORRECT ANSWER FOR QUESTIONS 11 TO 14 FROM CHOICES 1 THROUGH 5.

1. Coumadin   **2.** heparin

3. warfarin   **4.** prothrombin time (PT)

5. partial thromboplastin time (PTT)

11. Test that measures the effect of heparin therapy

12. Another name for Coumadin

13. Test that measures the effect of Coumadin therapy

14. Can be taken orally at home for anticoagulant therapy

SELECT THE CORRECT ANSWER FOR QUESTIONS 15 TO 21 FROM CHOICES 1 THROUGH 6:

1. lithium heparin   **4.** sodium citrate

2. potassium oxalate   **5.** sodium heparin

3. EDTA   **6.** clot activator

15. The following anticoagulants form calcium salts.

    _____ _____ _____

16. Anticoagulant used to preserve erythrocytes, leukocytes,

    and thrombocytes. _____

17. Anticoagulant that inactivates thrombin but is lethal to

    cells. _____

18. Anticoagulant used in tubes for karyotyping. _____

19. Anticoagulant(s) that inactivate thrombin activity.

    _____ _____

20. Anticoagulant with 1:9 ratio to blood specimen._____

21. Most plastic tubes have this ingredient _____.

TRUE OR FALSE

22. A bleeding time is a precise and accurate measurement of platelet function.

23. Thrombocytopenia means decreased number of platelets.

24. Petechiae are seen when a patient has thrombocytopenia.

25. A clot in a lavender-top tube results in an increased platelet count.

26. Poor platelet adhesiveness will result in a good platelet plug.

27. A platelet function assay is a quick screening measurement of platelet function.

ESSAY QUESTIONS

28. Explain why a discard tube is drawn before a blue-top tube. Explain why the order of filling different colored tubes may differ with a syringe versus a Vacutainer.

29. What is a blood thinner? Why is it prescribed? What precautions must the phlebotomist take?

30. Explain why the tube drawn for a PT or PTT must be full. Explain why two blue-top tubes that are partially full cannot be combined.

31. Explain why a blood sample for a karyotype requires a sodium heparin tube.

32. What is HIPAA? Why do phlebotomists need to be aware of HIPAA?

33. What is DIC? How does this condition affect the blood sample? What should the phlebotomist do if he or she encounters a patient or blood sample with this condition?

34. Explain why a syringe or Vacutainer may fill with blood very slowly. What may happen to the blood sample if this occurs?

Infection Control

CASE 16
Active Tuberculosis (TB)

Ms. C.B. is an 18-year-old woman hospitalized for active tuberculosis (TB) and is placed in a negative-pressure isolation room. She has begun treatment with isoniazid. Because there is some risk of liver toxicity on this medication, a liver panel and peak and trough blood samples for quantitation of isoniazid levels have been ordered. The liver panel and initial isoniazid level are ordered for 6 AM with a next isoniazid level to follow 8 hours later. The patient also has a history of IV drug use. Debbie is the phlebotomist responsible for the next timed-blood draw.

Key Words: acid-fast bacilli • airborne precautions • blood-borne pathogen • Centers for Disease Control and Prevention (CDC) • Hepatitis B (HBV) • HIV • Hospital Infection Control Practices Advisory Committee (HICPAC) • injection drug use • multidrug resistance • negative-pressure isolation room • N95 respirator • personal protective equipment (PPE) • respiratory infection • standard precautions • therapeutic drug monitoring • transmission-based precautions • tuberculosis

QUESTIONS

1. TB can be a nosocomial infection. What does this statement mean? How is the cocaine use related?

2. What infectious disease precautions do you need to observe with this patient?

3. What is a negative-pressure isolation room?

4. When does the next blood sample need to be drawn? Why is it important that it be drawn on time and the exact time recorded?

5. What difficulties should the phlebotomist be prepared for with this patient?

DISCUSSION OF CASE STUDY

1. TB is caused by *Mycobacterium tuberculosis* bacteria. *Mycobacterium* is also referred to as an acid-fast bacillus because of its characteristic reaction to certain stains. Staining reactions are used to identify bacteria, and in the case of TB, it is a slender red-staining rod when stained for its acid-fast reaction. TB is highly contagious because it is most commonly acquired as a respiratory air-borne infection. Furthermore, many strains of TB are highly resistant to antibiotics (multidrug resistant) and therefore are difficult to treat. *Mycobacterium* is very difficult to kill because it has a waxy coat that makes it resistant to drying, temperature changes, disinfectants, and normal body defense responses. TB organisms can remain alive for years inside a granuloma formation inside the lung. Consequently, once a patient has acquired a TB infection, a regular TB radiograph is necessary to ensure that the spot on the lung radiograph (granuloma) stays the same size and therefore inactive. TB can be acquired as a nosocomial infection, i.e., in the hospital. Hospital staff can be infected from a patient, or one patient can infect other patients. For this reason, Ms. C.B. has been placed in an isolation room.

   Ms. C.B. also has a history of cocaine use. She is likely to be an injection drug user and could be positive for hepatitis B (HBV) and HIV. Often, a patient's clinical history may not be available to the phlebotomist. It is possible to recognize drug injection lesions (needle track marks). A series of photocards, illustrating the appearance of skin lesions on injection drug users, is available free from the Substance Abuse and Mental Health Services Administration (SAMHSA) or the Center for Substance Abuse Treatment (CSAT). The Department of Health and Human Services (DHHS) publication number is (SMA) 02-3753. To obtain a copy of the photocards, the SAMHSA phone number is (800) 729-6686, or visit www.csat.samhsa.gov/.

2. TB is transmitted by being enclosed within droplet nuclei. Small droplets of mucus are generated by talking or sneezing. The liquid in these droplets evaporates into the air, but the organisms within the dried mucus remain viable and suspended in the air or in dust particles for long periods of time (Fig. 3.1).

   HBV and HIV are blood-borne pathogens. These are viruses that circulate in the blood and are commonly acquired as sexually transmitted diseases (STDs). As the phlebotomist, Debbie must be concerned with acquiring these diseases as an accidental needle stick or by blood or other body fluids entering through mucous membranes or through cuts or abrasions on the skin. To avoid occupational exposure and risk of infection, Debbie must observe CDC and HICPAC guidelines for isolation procedures in hospitals. These guidelines include Standard Precautions and Transmission-Based Precautions for airborne pathogens and blood-borne pathogens.

3. Ms. C.B. has been placed in a private isolation room with negative-pressure. This means that the air circulation and air pressure in the room are designed so that more air comes in than goes out. This decreases the chances of infectious microbes being spread into the adjoining corridor. The door to Ms. C.B.'s room should be closed at all times with a sign posted for appropriate precautions. A small room

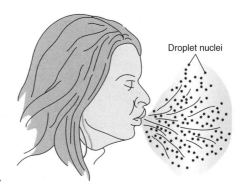

Figure 3.1.   Droplet Nuclei.

or cart with all supplies necessary to enter the room and for care of the patient should be outside the door. Debbie needs to gather exactly the supplies she needs for drawing Ms. C.B.'s blood sample. The tourniquet should be left in the room. A protective gown, gloves, goggles, and mask are necessary for entering Ms. C.B.'s room. Debbie needs an N95 respirator that has been fit-tested specifically for Debbie's use only (Fig. 3.2). This respirator has a special filter built into the mask to prevent airborne microbes from entering Debbie's respiratory system. Some states now require fit-testing to be performed yearly. A regular surgical mask is **not** sufficient protection against acquiring TB.

Debbie should review procedures for Standard Precautions and Transmission-Based Precautions so that she can draw Ms. C.B.'s blood specimen efficiently and safely.

4. Debbie needs to obtain a timed blood draw for therapeutic drug monitoring. For a drug to be effective and to avoid complications caused by drug toxicity, appropriate dosage levels must be monitored. The trough level is the lowest concentration of drug in the patient's serum, and the peak is the highest concentration. How rapidly a drug is absorbed varies with the type of drug and an individual patient's metabolism. The nursing staff, pharmacy, and physician all need to know what the peak and trough levels are to adjust dosage. They also need to know when the peak and trough values are reached. Thus Debbie, the phlebotomist, has a very important responsibility in drawing the blood sample when it is ordered and recording the exact time the sample is drawn. If an initial blood sample was drawn at 6 AM, the next blood sample needs to be drawn at 2 PM (Fig. 3.3).

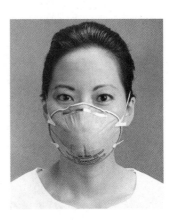

Figure 3.2.   N95 Respirator.

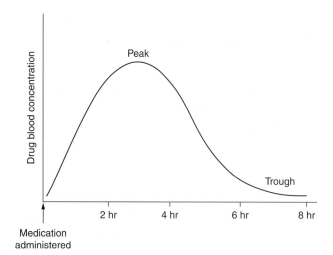

Figure 3.3. Therapeutic Drug Monitoring.

5. Not only does Debbie need to be concerned with isolation procedures and all of the infectious disease precautions, but also she
   needs to be aware of her patient's physical and emotional well-
   being. Ms. C.B. is a young woman who is or previously was an IV
   drug user. She might have emotional problems, depression, and may
   not be very cooperative. Debbie should not hesitate to ask for help
   if Ms. C.B. is unwilling or unable to lie still. With Ms. C.B.'s history
   of injection drug use, she may have veins that are sclerosed, scarred,
   and difficult to access for venipuncture. Debbie needs to be sure she
   has a 23-gauge butterfly needle blood collection set as a back-up, if
   Ms. C.B.'s veins are not accessible with a syringe or Vacutainer. Of
   course, Debbie must also observe safety precautions with self-
   sheathing needles and appropriate sharps disposal.

CASE 17
Accidental Needle Stick Injury

J.M. is a 26-year-old Hispanic man and is a known IV drug user. His
veins are badly sclerosed because of years of abuse. He needs an HIV
(human immunodeficiency virus) test, HBV (hepatitis B virus) test, and
HCV (hepatitis C virus) antibody test. Dennis, the phlebotomist, is able to
locate a vein in the hand on a second attempt using a butterfly. As
Dennis is withdrawing the needle, the patient suddenly jerks his hand.
Drops of blood spatter on Dennis's lab coat and he is accidentally stuck
in the finger by the needle.

Key Words: blood-borne pathogen • hepatitis B virus (HBV) • hepatitis
C virus (HCV) • human immunodeficiency virus (HIV) • needle stick
injury • polymerase chain reaction (PCR) • prophylaxis

QUESTIONS

1. What should be Dennis's immediate response?

2. What subsequent steps need to be taken?

3. What type of diseases do HIV and HCV cause? What are the initial symptoms? How are these diseases diagnosed?

4. Should Dennis be concerned about the blood on his lab coat?

DISCUSSION OF CASE STUDY

1. Dennis needs to immediately rinse any blood from the puncture site and apply an antiseptic such as povidone-iodine for at least 60 seconds. Fortunately, Dennis was wearing plastic safety glasses and there was no splatter of blood near his face. If any blood had splattered into Dennis's nose, eyes, or mouth and possible mucous membrane exposure had occurred, he would need to flush the site with water for a minimum of 10 minutes.

2. Dennis must report the accident to his supervisor. Dennis then needs to go immediately to a health care provider for evaluation, counseling, and possible treatment. Because the patient is a known IV drug user, there is a real possibility that he is HIV, HBV, and/or HCV positive. Blood from Dennis and the patient needs to be tested for these viral diseases. Hopefully, Dennis has been vaccinated for HBV and has an adequate antibody level. If the patient is positive for HIV, Dennis needs to have his blood tested for HIV immediately and at periodic intervals— normally 6 weeks, 12 weeks, 6 months, and 1 year after exposure. Dennis may be given azidothymidine (AZT) or another HIV medication to help prevent infection. Unfortunately, treatments for HCV are not as well developed as those for HIV.

3. HIV, HBV, and HCV are blood-borne pathogens. These viruses circulate in the blood and can be transmitted through contact with blood and body fluids. They are most likely acquired as STDs (sexually transmitted diseases), but can also be transmitted by drug addicts sharing needles or in accidents involving health care personnel. HIV kills T-helper lymphocytes. T-helper lymphocytes can be recognized by a surface membrane molecule called CD4 surfaces. HIV attaches to CD4 and as this lymphocyte population is eliminated, the body becomes susceptible to many diseases. Currently, with multiple drug treatments, it is possible to slow the process of T-helper lymphocyte death, but HIV will still be present in the body. Initial symptoms of HIV are much like the flu. These symptoms can then disappear, but the virus is multiplying, and as more CD4 lymphocytes are lost, eventually full-blown symptoms of AIDS appear. HIV is diagnosed by the presence of antibodies to HIV. Only if the virus is present will the patient's immune system form antibodies. Unfortunately, these antibodies are not protective. Once HIV is diagnosed, the levels of virus in the blood can be measured by a molecular test called polymerase chain reaction (PCR). Progression of AIDS is

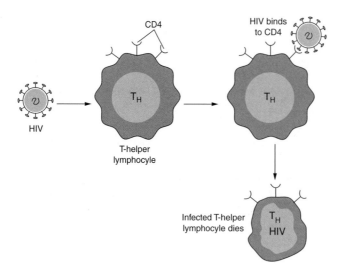

Figure 3.4. Anatomy of HIV Infection.

monitored by measuring the number of CD4 lymphocytes in the blood (Fig. 3.4).

HBV and HCV are viruses that attack the liver. Most health care workers are protected from HBV infection by vaccination. If not protected by vaccination, most individuals infected with HBV will develop acute hepatitis and then their immune systems will clear the infection. However, in a small number of patients, chronic liver infections can develop, which can lead to liver cancer. This same scenario is also true for hepatitis C. Unfortunately, no vaccine is available for HCV. Flu-like symptoms are also seen initially with HBV or HCV, although approximately 50% of infected individuals may not have symptoms. HBV or HCV infections are confirmed by detection of viral antigens in the blood.

4. Dennis does not need to be too concerned about the blood on his lab coat. Rinsing with 10% bleach should inactivate the virus. Likewise, any blood on the floor should be absorbed with paper towels soaked with 10% bleach. Paper towels should be disposed in an appropriate container (Fig. 3.5).

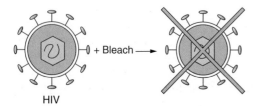

Figure 3.5. Bleach Kills HIV.

CASE 18
Urine Spill

Ms. P.D. is a 16-year-old woman who entered an outpatient clinic with complaints of abdominal cramps and vaginal bleeding. She had no nausea or vomiting. The pain had increased in the previous 24 hours, and at the time of examination she also complained of pain in the upper right abdominal quadrant. The physician has ordered a stat complete blood count (CBC) and urinalysis. The blood is drawn with no problem. Because this is stat, Melissa, the phlebotomist, delivered the blood and urine to the laboratory. On the way to the laboratory, Melissa noticed that the lid of the urine sample was loose and some urine had spilled into a compartment in her tray.

Key Words: *Chlamydia* • disinfectant • PID • specimen transportation • urine contamination

QUESTIONS

1. Is the urine sample still useful for testing purposes? How should the urine sample have been correctly handled and transported? What kinds of transportation alternatives are available?

2. How should Melissa clean the spill? What kind of microbes does she need to be concerned about?

DISCUSSION OF CASE STUDY

1. The urine sample is probably still useful for testing purposes. Of course when Melissa placed identifying labels on the sample she should have also checked the lid to ensure that it was secure. She also could have placed the urine container inside of a plastic sealable bag. If this specimen were being transported via a pneumatic tube system, a protective biohazard plastic bag would have been a must to prevent contamination of the system by leaks or breakages of containers. If the blood tubes were also contaminated by the urine sample, the outsides of the tubes would need to be disinfected with 10% bleach and identifying labels replaced.

2. Melissa will have to clean and dispose of any equipment and supplies that may have been contaminated by the urine spill. It would probably be a good idea to rinse and wipe out her tray with 10% bleach to disinfect thoroughly. There are many bacteria, fungi, and even protozoa that are potential pathogens in urine. *Chlamydia*, which causes pelvic inflammatory disease (PID), is the most common female reproductive tract infection. This disease is acquired as a sexually transmitted disease (STD). If Melissa observes Standard Precautions and has disinfected her tray thoroughly, she need not worry.

CASE 19
Blood Cultures

D.M. is a 53-year-old man with a history of Guillain-Barré syndrome
and septicemia with methicillin-resistant *Staphylococcus aureus*,
vancomycin-resistant *Enterococcus facium*, and *Pseudomonas aeruginosa*.
At the rehabilitation hospital, the patient complained of shortness of
breath and tachycardia. He had a temperature of 102°F. He also had an
indwelling Foley catheter. Two sets of blood cultures have been ordered
6 hours apart. Lucinda is the phlebotomist who must draw the first set
of blood cultures.

Key Words: *Enterococcus* (VRE) • Foley catheter • methicillin-resistant
Staphylococcus aureus (MRSA) • normal flora septicemia • timed blood
culture • vancomycin

QUESTIONS

1. What is an MRSA? What is the significance of vancomycin-resistant
   enterococci?

2. What is meant by a blood culture set? Why are two sets of blood cultures ordered? What is the optimum amount of blood to be collected?

3. How is a blood culture obtained? Explain the procedure and the reasons
   for each step.

4. Are any special precautions necessary? Is the presence of an indwelling
   Foley catheter significant?

DISCUSSION OF CASE STUDY

1. Mr. D.M. has a history of several dangerous bacterial infections. Each
   of the organisms listed is a dangerous pathogen by itself, but what
   makes them even more dangerous is that they have been identified as
   antibiotic resistant. Methicillin-resistant *Staphylococcus aureus*
   (MRSA) is a strain of *Staphylococcus* resistant to all penicillin-related
   antibiotics. Once infection with MRSA is acquired, this infection is
   almost impossible to treat. One of the few effective antibiotics for treating MRSA is vancomycin. Mr. D.M. has also been infected with
   vancomycin-resistant *Enterococcus* (VRE). The ability to resist the
   effects of antibiotics is carried on bacterial genes. These genes can
   spread from one bacterial species to another. It is possible that Mr.
   D.M. became reinfected by the same organisms and that they all have
   become resistant to vancomycin. Mr. D.M. also has Guillain-Barré syndrome. This is a neurological disease characterized initially by a fever
   and then pain, weakness, and paralysis of muscles. Because of this dis-
   abling disease, Mr. D.M. is more susceptible to infection.

   To determine whether Mr. D.M. has reoccurrence of his previous
   infections and septicemia (bacteria circulating in the blood), blood
   cultures have been ordered. As the term implies, a blood sample from
   a patient is added to sterile bacterial growth medium. If bacteria grow

in the blood culture, they can be identified and their susceptibility to antibiotics can be tested (antibiotic susceptibility).

2. A set of blood cultures includes two bottles. One bottle is aerobic, and the other anaerobic. A blood sample and air are added to the aerobic culture bottle to encourage growth of bacteria that require oxygen (O_2). *Staphylococcus aureus* is an aerobic bacterium. The anaerobic bottle must be handled so that air is **not** introduced. Enterococci can sometimes grow better in anaerobic conditions. Two sets of blood cultures are ordered at two different times to enhance the probability of obtaining blood samples with circulating bacteria present.

  It is essential that the blood culture bottles be filled correctly. If Lucinda underfills, i.e., does not add enough blood to the blood culture bottles, she will decrease the chances of detecting circulating bacteria or it will take longer to detect the smaller number of bacteria present.

  What should Lucinda do if she is only able to obtain 10 mL of blood from the patient? (Adult blood culture bottles require 8 to 10 mL, pediatric bottles require 1 to 3 mL). Should Lucinda divide the 10 mL and place 5 mL of blood into each bottle? The better procedure would be to fill the aerobic bottle with 10 mL so that at least one bottle is full and the microbiology laboratory will have a better chance of detecting the bacteremia. She should fill the aerobic bottle because most pathogenic bacteria capable of causing a bacteremia will grow under aerobic conditions.

  Overfilling the blood culture bottle is also **not** useful. To aid the growth of the bacteria that may be present, the blood culture bottles are placed into an incubator at body temperature. Automated blood culture incubators detect bacterial growth by measuring the level of carbon dioxide (CO_2) in each bottle. With excess blood in the bottle, white blood cells can contribute CO_2 as well, and a blood culture bottle then appears to be positive for bacterial growth when it actually is not. The microbiologist wastes supplies and time trying to isolate and identify bacteria that are not there.

3. The procedures for obtaining a blood culture are designed to prevent contamination of the blood culture by normal flora on the skin or other bacteria not in the blood sample. Normal flora are the bacteria normally present that inhabit the skin. A good example is *Staphylococcus epidermidis*. *Staphylococcus epidermidis* is an organism similar to *Staphylococcus aureus*. However, *Staphylococcus epidermidis* is not generally a pathogen. It can contaminate a blood culture specimen, which may result in a true pathogen being missed, and time and supplies being wasted to identify a normal flora organism. Lucinda should carefully review her phlebotomy text for detailed procedures and consult with her supervisor for specific details for her work place site. A summary of steps and the reason for each step are presented below:

   • Lucinda should gather all necessary equipment and supplies and have them conveniently located next to the patient. This includes supplies for the venipuncture and specific supplies for the blood culture. Lucinda needs to have everything readily available so that once the venipuncture site is prepared the chances for contamination are decreased.

   • An appropriate vein is identified, and the site is prepared. First an alcohol swab is used to remove excess dirt. Lucinda should start in the center of the area to be cleansed, and with a circular motion,

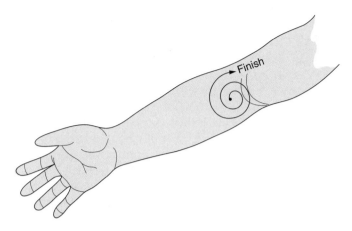

Figure 3.6. Preparing Arm for Blood Culture.

work outward. The site is then cleansed with a fresh iodine swab (povidone-iodine or iodine tincture), beginning in the center and rubbing outward in concentric circles. Lucinda should not go back over any area that has previously been covered to prevent contamination of a previously cleaned site. The area is allowed to air dry for 30 to 60 seconds to ensure effective antiseptic action. Chlorhexidine and alcohol solution may be used in place of alcohol and iodine (Fig. 3.6).

- Lucinda should then prepare the blood culture vials. The protective cover is removed, and the tops of the vials are wiped with a fresh alcohol swab. The vials are not sterile on the outside. The alcohol removes the iodine. If iodine enters the blood culture vial, it can inhibit bacterial growth. Some manufacturers recommend using only alcohol for wiping the tops of blood culture vials. The alcohol wipe is removed, and the rubber stopper is allowed to dry. Once the rubber stopper is cleaned, it cannot be touched.

- Lucinda is now ready to perform the venipuncture. She should not repalpate the sterilized site with her gloved finger unless sterile gloves are used or the gloved finger is decontaminated with alcohol or chlorhexidine.

- The blood sample can be transferred into the blood culture vials directly if using a Vacutainer safety holder and needle device. If using a syringe or butterfly, a sterile adapter may be necessary for transferring the blood into the blood culture bottle or vial. If the blood sample is drawn into a syringe, the blood is delivered first into the anaerobic vial and then the aerobic vial. With a butterfly, the blood is delivered into the aerobic vial first because the tubing will contain air. The anaerobic vial is then filled.

  Note: Blood culture collection methods can differ slightly among laboratories.

4. With Mr. D.M.'s history of an MRSA, Lucinda should be aware of contact infection disease precautions. She should be wearing PPE (laboratory coat, gloves). She needs to wash her hands before and after contacting the patient. Mr. D.M.'s Foley catheter is not an issue in this case. He probably needs the catheter inserted into the bladder because of his muscle paralysis and mobility problems. The Foley catheter drains urine directly into an attached bag. Lucinda should be aware that these catheters readily become contaminated with bacteria and urinary tract infections are the most common type of nosocomial (hospital acquired) infection.

CASE 20
Reverse Isolation

Mrs. C.L. is a 58-year-old woman who has recently undergone a bone marrow transplantation. She is recovering and is presently in reverse isolation. Her physician has ordered a complete blood count (CBC).

Key Words: bone marrow transplantation • embryonic stem cells • hematopoietic stem cells • immune susceptibility • metastatic cancer • reverse isolation

QUESTIONS

1. What is reverse isolation? Why is reverse isolation indicated? What precautions need to be taken with reverse isolation?

2. Why is Mrs. C.L. in reverse isolation?

3. What is a bone marrow transplantation?

DISCUSSION OF CASE STUDY

1. Reverse isolation is protective isolation. Mrs. C.L. does not have an infection, but she is highly vulnerable to infection, and with her present condition an infection could be fatal. Therefore she is in isolation in a private room to **protect** her from infection. Signs have been posted indicating reverse isolation and the special precautions to be taken. These precautions are similar to other isolation procedures. Good hand washing technique and gowns, gloves, and masks are usually necessary to prevent the patient from acquiring any infection. Blood samples and other articles taken out of the room do not need to be double bagged because these patients do not have infection; however, articles entering the room must be sterile or carefully decontaminated.

2. Mrs. C.L. is in reverse isolation because she has recently undergone a bone marrow transplantation.

3. A bone marrow transplantation is the replacement of a patient's bone marrow. Bone marrow transplantations are performed when the patient's own bone marrow is defective or if cancerous cells are present. The bone marrow is the source of blood cells. Within the bone marrow are hematopoietic stem cells. Stem cells are cells that have the ability to proliferate and develop into many different types of cells. Embryonic stem cells are derived from embryos and have the ability to develop into any cell type found in the body. Hematopoietic stem cells (HSC) have the ability to

develop into the various blood cell types. HSCs can become diseased and fail to develop into mature blood cells. HSCs can become mutated and develop into a leukemia. Cancer cells from other parts of the body can invade the bone marrow and begin to grow (metastatic cancer). In the case of leukemia or metastatic cancer of the bone marrow, chemotherapy (various types of drugs) may be used to help suppress or kill the cancer cell. Another mode of treatment is a bone marrow transplantation.

A bone marrow transplantation is a very dangerous and complex procedure. As with all organ transplantations, an appropriately matched donor must be found or the transplant will be rejected. The patient's diseased marrow must be eliminated either by radiation treatment or by toxic drugs. Donor marrow is then infused into the patient. The donor marrow must be accepted by the patient's immune system. It is also possible for the donor marrow to reject the patient's tissues. If rejection does not occur, the donor marrow adapts to its new home and will begin making new blood cells.

Before the formation of new blood cells by the donor marrow, the patient has no ability to form new white blood cells. Should the patient acquire an infection, there are no white blood cells to fight bacteria or stimulate a good immune response. These patients are highly susceptible to infection and thus are placed in reverse isolation.

CASE 21
Staphylococcus Aureus

Mr. H.M. is a 37-year-old white man hospitalized for multiple fractures in the left hip because of a work-related accident. He recently had surgery to correct the fractures. Sharing the same room is patient Mr. P.R., who has recently undergone abdominal surgery. Mr. P.R. has just been identified with a *Staphylococcus aureus* (SA) infection in the wound site and is waiting to be moved to a private room. Mr. H.M. needs a complete blood count (CBC) and protime (PT). Mr. P.R. also needs blood drawn for a CBC. Priscilla is the phlebotomist who is to draw the blood sample from MR. H.M. and MR. P.R.

Key Words: abdominal surgery • bone/wound infections • Contact Precautions • orthopedic surgery • PPE • Standard Precautions • *Staph. aureus*

QUESTIONS

1. Are there special precautions Priscilla must observe in drawing blood from these patients?

2. What procedures must be observed?

DISCUSSION OF CASE STUDY

1. There are definitely special precautions Priscilla must observe in drawing blood from Mr. H.M. and Mr. P.R. Mr. P.R. recently had abdominal surgery and has already been identified as having an SA infection in his surgical

wound site. SA is a bacterium capable of causing severe infections and complications. It is now a bacterium that is frequently resistant to methicillin-type antibiotics (penicillin), making it a difficult bacterial infection to treat.

Mr. H.M. has recently undergone orthopedic surgery to correct a fractured hip. Fracture of the hip involves one of the largest bones in the body, the femur. Hip surgery is complex, and a considerable amount of blood loss can occur, requiring blood transfusions. Mr. H.M. probably has a large wound site. If surgery is successful and no complications occur, the bone heals quite well. However, if infection occurs, the bone may not heal and Mr. H.M. will have a very painful and long recovery. SA is notorious as a dangerous infection of bone. These two patients should not be in the same room because of the danger of SA being spread from Mr. P.R. to Mr. H.M. However, this is not a decision that Priscilla has responsibility for. Priscilla does have a responsibility to ensure, as much as possible, that she does not carry SA from one patient to another. Should Mr. H.M. acquire an SA infection from Mr. P.R., legal action could be taken.

2. Priscilla has been informed that Mr. P.R. has SA; it would be better to draw Mr. H.M. first. This would decrease the possibilities of Mr. H.M. contracting SA from Mr. P.R. SA is a bacterium spread mostly by contact. Standard Precautions and Contact Precautions should be observed. Priscilla should wear personal protective equipment (PPE). Good hand washing technique is essential before and after coming into contact with each patient, which means removing gloves and replacing with fresh gloves and washing her hands thoroughly. Likewise, she should remove her gloves before leaving the patients' room so as not to contaminate subsequent patients (Fig. 3.7).

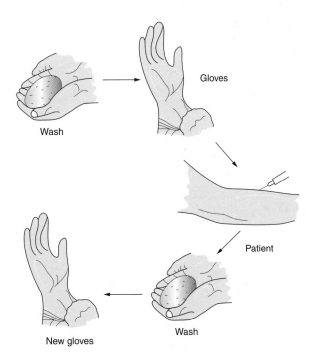

Figure 3.7. Washing Hands and Using New Gloves.

Quiz

MULTIPLE CHOICE

1. Important characteristics of *Mycobacterium tuberculosis* include ____.
   a. also called acid-fast because of its staining reaction
   b. highly resistant to disinfectants
   c. easily killed by lung macrophages
   d. a and b
   e. a, b, and c

2. What does it mean if a person has a positive TB skin test result?
   a. The person has TB.
   b. The person had TB.
   c. The person may have had a subclinical infection and now tests positive.
   d. a and b
   e. a, b, and c

3. PPE necessary when drawing blood from a TB-positive patient includes gloves, goggles, and ____.
   a. N95 respirator
   b. N95 respirator, fit-tested
   c. surgical mask
   d. face shield
   e. surgical shoe coverings

4. Steps to be taken with an accidental needle stick are ____.
   a. rinse blood from puncture site
   b. apply antiseptic
   c. report accident to supervisor
   d. see health care provider for possible prophylactic treatment
   e. all of the above

5. Vaccines are available for ____
   a. HBV
   b. HSV
   c. HIV
   d. HCV
   e. CMV

6. HIV is diagnosed by _____.
   a. loss of CD4 lymphocytes
   b. presence of viral particles
   c. presence of antibodies to HIV
   d. loss of CD8 lymphocytes
   e. presence of viral cDNA

7. If blood or urine samples are transported to the laboratory via a pneumatic tube system, samples must ____.
   a. be labeled correctly
   b. be placed in a protective biohazard plastic bag
   c. be wiped with bleach
   d. a and b
   e. a, b, and c

8. The minimal concentration of bleach for disinfection is _____.
   a. 0.5%
   b. 1%
   c. 5%
   d. 10%
   e. 100%

9. A septicemia is an _____.
   a. infection of the urinary tract
   b. infection of the blood
   c. infection of the sinuses
   d. infection of the inner ear
   e. infection of the lung

10. Which of the following is an aerobic bacteria?
   a. *Staphylococcus aureus*
   b. *Mycobacterium tuberculosae*
   c. enterococci
   d. a and b
   e. a, b, and c

11. If using a butterfly needle apparatus to draw a blood culture set and a
   CBC, which tube or vial is drawn first?
   a. lavender-top tube
   b. aerobic blood culture bottle
   c. anaerobic blood culture bottle
   d. red-top tube
   e. black-top tube

12. Which statement is *incorrect* concerning normal flora of the skin?
    a. normal flora refers to bacteria normally present
    b. *Staph. aureus* is part of the normal flora of the skin
    c. *Staph. epidermidis* is part of the normal flora of the skin
    d. a and b
    e. a and c

13. When cleansing a site for blood culture, which of the following statements is *not* true?
    a. An alcohol swab is used first, followed by iodine.
    b. A circular motion beginning in the center and moving outward is used to clean the site.
    c. A previously cleaned area should not be retouched.
    d. After cleansing, the vein may be repalpated with a gloved finger.

14. If not enough blood is added to a blood culture bottle _____.
    a. the probability of detecting bacteria is decreased
    b. it may take longer to detect whether bacteria are present in the patient's blood
    c. carbon dioxide levels become increased
    d. a and b
    e. a, b, and c

15. Blood culture bottles with the appropriate amount of blood in them are placed in _____ at _____ temperature.
    a. incubator . . . room
    b. incubator . . . body
    c. microbiology . . . room
    d. hematology . . . room

16. The most common type of nosocomial infection is ___.
    a. urinary tract
    b. respiratory
    c. skin
    d. surgical wounds
    e. neonatal

17. A patient in reverse isolation _____.
    a. has a very dangerous contagious infection
    b. is highly vulnerable to infection
    c. may have a suppressed immune system
    d. a and b
    e. b and c

18. Hematopoietic stem cells _____.

    a. have the ability to develop into any cell type of the body

    b. have the ability to form all types of blood cells

    c. are found in the bone marrow

    d. a and b

    e. b and c

19. An MRSA _____.

    a. is a bacteria that is not inhibited by routine antibiotics

    b. can cause serious bone infections

    c. can cause serious wound infections

    d. is spread mostly by contact

    e. all of the above

MATCHING
Match the microorganism with the transmission mode.

20. HBV	a. STD
21. HIV	b. injection drug use
22. TB	c. contact
23. *Staphylococcus aureus*	d. droplet nuclei
	e. a and b

MATCH THE ACRONYM WITH THE DESCRIPTION:

24. AZT	a. protective goggles
25. PPE	b. cell receptor for HIV
26. CDC	c. metastatic cancer cell
27. CD4	d. government agency that monitors disease
	e. therapeutic drug for HIV

ESSAY QUESTIONS

28. Explain why it is important to draw a blood sample at a precise time for therapeutic drug monitoring.

29. Explain how phlebotomists may avoid risks with blood-borne pathogens such as HBV or HIV.

30. Why is a methicillin-resistant *Staph. aureus* infection so dangerous?

31. Why are two sets of blood cultures at two different times often ordered for a patient with suspected septicemia?

32. Explain why blood culture bottles should not be overfilled or underfilled.

33. Outline the necessary steps in drawing a blood culture to ensure that no contamination occurs.

Complex Patient and Environmental Factors in Quality Specimen Collection

CASE 22
Antibiotic Toxicity/Therapeutic Dose Monitoring

Pseudomonas aeruginosa was cultured in Mrs. S.W.'s sputum 2 months ago, and now a sinus culture for her was found to be positive for *Pseudomonas*. The organism showed antibiotic sensitivity to gentamicin, ciprofloxacin, and aztreonam. Mrs. S.W. stated she was allergic to ciprofloxacin. Mrs. S.W. was therefore prescribed gentamicin (400 mg every 24 hours). Peak and trough blood levels for gentamicin were ordered, as well as creatinine tests. Because gentamicin can be toxic to the kidneys and auditory nerves, blood for creatinine tests was to be drawn at the same time.

Mrs. S.W.'s initial creatinine level was 1.0 mg/dL (normal levels, creatinine = 0.7 to 1.3 mg/dL). The blood was to be drawn for peak gentamicin level 30 minutes postinfusion and trough levels 30 minutes before the patient was given the antibiotic.

After 48 hours, Mrs. S.W.'s creatinine was 1.1 mg/dL with a gentamicin trough of 2.3 (normal gentamicin trough for this dosing regimen 0 to 0.5). Therefore, gentamicin was discontinued for 48 hours. After this time period, the gentamicin trough was <0.3, and Mrs. S.W. was again administered a dose of gentamicin. 48 hours later the gentamicin trough was 4.5 and creatinine 1.7. Sam was the early morning phlebotomist who drew this last trough specimen. However, he neglected to label this sample with the correct time and whether the sample was a trough, peak, or random sample. Because the sample was not labeled properly, it was erroneously assumed to be a random sample and the physician was not notified. Test results were not reviewed for Mrs. S.W. by the pharmacist and physician until 48 hours later. At this time Mrs. S.W. complained of dizziness, ringing in the ears, and problems with balance, and the gentamicin was discontinued.

Key Words: antibiotic sensitivity • antibiotic toxicity • negligence
• *Pseudomonas aeruginosa* • timed blood draws • therapeutic drug
monitoring

QUESTIONS

1. What is *Pseudomonas?*

2. What went wrong?

3. How is the phlebotomist involved?

4. Is this a case for litigation?

DISCUSSION OF CASE STUDY

1. *Pseudomonas aeruginosa* is a gram-negative bacteria commonly present in soil and water. It is highly resistant to soaps, disinfectants, drying, and temperature extremes and is a frequent contaminant of ventilators, intravenous solutions, hospital instruments, and utensils. It is an opportunistic organism, i.e., it can cause severe infections in individuals with depressed immune systems. It is also resistant to many commonly used antibiotics. An antibiotic sensitivity test to determine which antibiotics are effective against this organism is very important for treatment of this patient.

2. The initial creatinine level for Mrs. S.W. was within normal range. However, it quickly became elevated, and likewise the trough level for gentamicin did not decrease to within an acceptable range. Mrs. S.W. was evidently experiencing antibiotic toxicity by the time the most recent laboratory test results were reviewed.

Therapeutic drug monitoring is a complex procedure that involves careful coordination and communication between the laboratory, the pharmacy, and the patient's physician. Gentamicin is an effective antibiotic; however, it can be toxic, and appropriate dosage levels must be carefully monitored. To adequately evaluate dosage, accurate collection of trough and peak blood samples is imperative. Trough levels in the blood indicate when the drug concentration is lowest, and collection of blood samples should occur just before administration of the drug. Sam, the phlebotomist, collected the trough sample, but failed to label the sample properly. In the meantime, Mrs. S.W. was administered another dose of gentamicin even though her creatinine level was elevated (Figs. 4.1 and 4.2).

3. Signs of drug toxicity have definitely occurred as a result of negligence by not only Sam, but also the nursing staff, the pharmacy, and the attending physician. Results of previous creatinine tests showed elevated levels. The most recent test results should have been immediately brought to the attention of the nursing staff by the laboratory. Nursing should have then notified Mrs. S.W.'s physician. Nursing staff and pharmacy personnel should have been monitoring these values before administering another dose of gentamicin. The phlebotomist failed to label the trough sample correctly and caused a delay in the test results getting to the physician. Mrs. S.W. has valid justification for filing a law suit against the hospital and numerous departments and personnel.

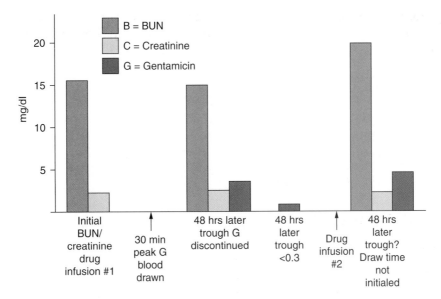

Figure 4.1.   Therapeutic Drug Monitoring, Example 1.

4. This is a case for litigation. Quality assurance step-by-step procedures and instructions for collecting timed-draw blood samples need to be established and adhered to. Lines of communication for all personnel who need to be alerted to drug levels and other test information need to be known and followed. This information needs to be relayed to appropriate parties in a timely manner. The phlebotomist has a critical role in drug monitoring. Sam is guilty of negligence, and disciplinary action may be taken against Sam for not properly labeling Mrs. S.W.'s blood sample.

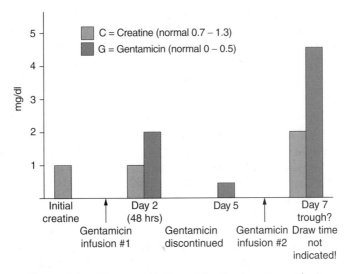

Figure 4.2.   Therapeutic Drug Monitoring, Example 2.

CASE 23
Patient Identification

Diana is one of the phlebotomists in an outpatient blood-drawing center. It has been a very busy day. It is now 6 PM and only one patient remains. Diana has a requisition for a Mrs. Jane Smith for a CBC and glucose. Diana is very tired and must leave to pick up her child at the child-care facility. The patient is an elderly woman who is sitting in the waiting room reading a magazine. Diana tells the woman, "Oh, you must be Mrs. Smith, my last patient." Diana then leads the woman to a blood-drawing chair. The patient is a difficult draw and requires two attempts to obtain the blood sample. Five minutes later, a younger woman comes into the blood drawing center and tells the receptionist she is Mrs. Jane Smith.

Key Words: geriatrics • patient identification

QUESTIONS

1. What errors did Diana commit?

2. How should patient identification be established?

3. What considerations in working with geriatric patients need to be considered?

DISCUSSION OF CASE STUDY

1. Diana did not correctly establish the identification of her patient. She assumed that the woman sitting in the waiting area was Mrs. Smith. Nor did Diana ask for any information from the elderly lady to confirm her identity.

2. Correct procedure to establish identification is to first ask the patient for his or her name. Diana should *not* have asked if the patient was Mrs. Smith. The elderly woman may not have good hearing and she could have Alzheimer disease. She may indeed be Mrs. Smith, but the mother of the younger Mrs. Smith and simply waiting for her daughter to pick her up. Therefore, not only should the name be correctly identified, but also date of birth or a patient identification number or an ID card should be checked to verify that the correct patient's blood is being drawn. For a hospital to currently maintain JACHO accreditation, Diana must verify patient identification with at least two separate pieces of information (Fig. 4.3).

3. The elderly or geriatric population constitutes a significant proportion of the patients seen by phlebotomists, and this population will continue to grow as the "baby boomers" age. Both physical disabilities and emotional and mental problems can occur with age. Hearing loss occurs commonly, and the elderly lady in this case may not have heard Diana correctly and was too embarrassed to ask Diana to repeat the name. As a phlebotomist working with an elderly patient, you may need to repeat instructions, speak louder, speak more slowly, and perhaps adjust your position so that you are speaking into the patient's "good ear."

Check ID

1. Ask patient name

2. Check ID bracelet

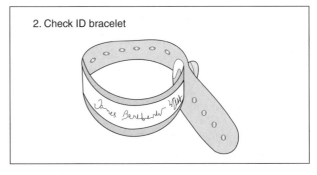

3. Check driver's license

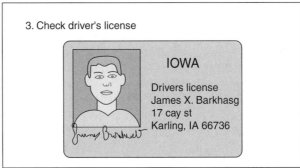

IOWA

Drivers license
James X. Barkhasg
17 cay st
Karling, IA 66736

Figure 4.3.   Verifying ID.

Even patients with hearing aids may have difficulty understanding you, since the hearing aid amplifies all sounds, including background noise. Elderly patients may also have arthritis or poor eyesight and need help sitting in the phlebotomy chair and getting up.

With age, the skin and underlying subcutaneous tissue become thinner. Muscles may atrophy. There is less support for veins, and the veins tend to "roll." If the skin is held extra-taut, this can help to hold the veins in place. A more shallow, smaller needle angle may be necessary for venipuncture.

Elderly patients may also be experiencing anger or depression from loss of a spouse, other family members, close friends, or loss of career and mobility. The phlebotomist should approach an elderly patient with patience, understanding, and compassion and address the patient with dignity and respect.

CASE 24
Dehydration

Patient T.M., a 28-year-old white man, enters the blood drawing center at 10 AM and tells the phlebotomist he had a terrible night. He was up several times vomiting, and the nurse in the doctor's office just told him he has a slight fever. The physician has ordered electrolytes, a liver panel, a CBC, and a serum iron level.

Key Words: dehydration • diurnal rhythms • effect of vomiting • electrolytes • pH • serum Fe

QUESTIONS

1. Is the patient likely to be dehydrated? Will this affect blood results? How?

2. Is it important to record at what time the blood is drawn? Why?

3. What tubes are necessary for these tests? Is order of draw important?

DISCUSSION OF CASE STUDY

1. As soon as the patient tells the phlebotomist he has been vomiting, a warning bell should go off. Vomiting can cause dehydration and loss of stomach acid (hydrochloric acid or HCl). Loss of water because of vomiting can affect blood volume and, because blood chemistry and CBC results are reported as amount of substance per deciliter, the liver panel and CBC results may be inaccurate. Loss of hydrochloric acid can affect blood pH values (acidity and alkalinity) and the electrolyte levels. Electrolytes routinely measured in a blood sample include sodium (Na^+), potassium (K^+), and chloride (Cl^-). Therefore, as a result of dehydration, CBC and liver panel values are likely to be slightly elevated and chloride levels may be decreased. Sodium and potassium levels are also likely to be abnormal if the patient has been sweating throughout the night because of fever and chills. A notation on the order form as to the patient's condition would be highly useful to the medical technologist and clinician as they attempt to evaluate the laboratory results.

2. A serum iron level (Fe) also has been ordered for this patient. Serum iron, along with certain hormones such as cortisol, adrenocorticotropic hormone (ACTH), thyroxin (T4), rennin, aldosterone, and insulin, are known to fluctuate with body diurnal rhythms. Body fluids also fluctuate according to the time of day. Thus it is very important to record the time the blood sample is drawn to aid the clinician in evaluating this patient's laboratory results.

   This patient is also likely to be experiencing inflammation because he has a fever. The patient's WBC count may be elevated. Should the patient need a follow-up CBC, it would be useful for the physician to know as accurately as possible when the previous blood sample was drawn to compare any changes over time in the WBC count or other blood values.

3. Electrolytes and the liver panel are most easily performed using a green-top lithium heparin tube. Be sure that a sodium heparin tube is *not* used, because the sodium in the anticoagulant of this tube will add to the sodium levels of the blood sample. The serum iron requires a red-top or gold-top tube. The polymer gel material in the gold-top or speckled serum separator tubes (SST) should not interfere with the iron components being tested. The CBC requires a lavender-top tube

containing EDTA. The order in which samples are drawn is important to ensure that anticoagulants do not contaminate subsequent tubes. If using a Vacutainer, the gold-top tube is drawn first, followed by green and then lavender tops. If using a syringe, a safety syringe transfer device should be used.

According to the NCCLS, the order of filling the evacuated tubes is the same. Some institutions prefer to reverse the order of filling when transferring from a syringe. The alternate order of filling assumes that blood entering the syringe last is the least likely to contain microclot formation. Sterile specimens are filled first, followed by anticoagulant tubes, then additive tubes, and finally non-additive tubes.

Care should be taken to prevent carryover or cross-contamination of additive from one tube to the next (Box 4.1). This can occur when the stopper puncturing needle or syringe transfer device needle comes into contact with blood in the tube. Blood remaining on or in the needle can be transferred to the next tube being filled. This process can be minimized by filling the tubes from the bottom up, as illustrated in Figure 4.4.

BOX 4.1

COMMON TESTS AFFECTED BY ADDITIVE CONTAMINATION

Tests Affected by Ethylenediaminetetraacetic Acid Contamination
  Calcium
  Partial thromboplastin
  Potassium
  Protime
  Serum iron
  Sodium
Tests Affected by Heparin Contamination
  Activated clotting time
  Partial thromboplastin
  Protime
Tests Affected by Potassium Oxalate Contamination
  Partial thromboplastin
  Potassium
  Protime
  Red cell morphology

Reprinted with permission from McCall RE, Tankersley CM. Phlebotomy Essentials. 3rd Ed. Philadelphia: Lippincott Williams & Wilkins, 2003.

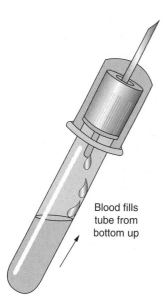

Blood fills
tube from
bottom up

Figure 4.4. Correct Method for Filling Tubes.

CASE 25
Renal and Liver Disease

Mr. T.R. is an elderly man who is hospitalized with cirrhosis and renal disease. A BUN, creatinine, liver panel, and ammonia are ordered for the patient. Mr. T.R. appears to be a bit restless and disoriented and does not readily respond to questions asked by the phlebotomist.

Key Words: ammonia • bleeding • cirrhosis • clotting factors • disorientation • ice slurry

QUESTIONS

1. What tubes are needed for these tests?

2. What special precautions need to be taken with these blood samples?

3. What special precautions need to be observed with this patient?

DISCUSSION OF CASE STUDY

1. The BUN, creatinine, and liver panel can all be drawn into a gold-top SST tubes. Depending on the procedures used in the laboratory, 5 to 10 mL of whole blood may need to be drawn. The ammonia needs to be drawn into a green-top heparin tube. Sodium or lithium heparin may be used.

2. The blood sample for the ammonia test needs to be specially handled. Ammonia is a blood component that rapidly breaks down, and to ensure accurate test results the green-top tube must be transported in an ice slurry. An ice slurry is a cup or plastic bag containing ice chips and water. The presence of the water ensures even distribution of the cold temperature throughout the blood sample. Submersion of the

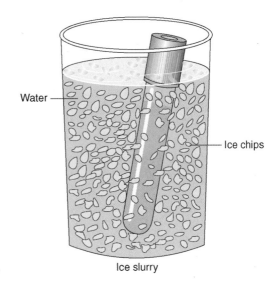

Water

Ice chips

Figure 4.5.   Blood Sample in Ice Slurry.   Ice slurry

blood sample tube into ice alone will result in a cold temperature where the ice touches the tube, but warmer spots where only air touches the tube. Sites where ice is in contact with the sides of the tube may also cause freezing of the RBCs. Subsequent thawing of the blood sample will result in hemolysis and an unacceptable blood sample (Fig. 4.5).

3. Blood urea nitrogen (BUN) and creatinine are waste products that are normally cleared by the kidney. With kidney disease or renal failure, these compounds will accumulate in the blood. Measuring the blood levels will indicate the severity of kidney damage. The liver panel and ammonia will assess liver function. In cirrhosis, ammonia accumulates in the blood and excessive levels will lead to mental disorientation. Mr. T.R. is likely suffering from disorientation caused by excessive ammonia levels. Mr. T.R. may not understand that blood tests have been ordered by his doctor and that you need to draw a blood sample. If he is moving about and likely will not lie still, you as the phlebotomist need to consult with the nursing station so that the nurse in charge of Mr. T.R. can speak with him, calm him, and hold his arm while the blood specimen is obtained.

   Because Mr. T.R. has liver disease and the liver is the major site for production of most of the clotting factors, it is likely that Mr. T.R. will bleed more readily after venipuncture. You or the nurse in charge of Mr. T.R.'s care will need to apply pressure at the venipuncture site for an additional length of time to ensure that he does not bruise or form a hematoma.

CASE 26
Home Health Care

Dave is a home health-care phlebotomist. He has been working two jobs, was out late the previous evening, overslept, and is a bit late to begin his morning pick-ups. He throws his tray in the car and heads out. His first patient is Mrs. P.S., a very thin elderly woman. She needs a PT and elec-trolyte panel. Dave's first attempt in the antecubital area is unsuccessful. He then decides to use a butterfly with a Vacutainer attachment on a hand vein. He places the tourniquet on the patient's arm just above the hand and selects the venipuncture site. He assembles his equipment and tubes, cleans the venipuncture site, and enters a hand vein. The blood flows very slowly into a 4-mL green-top tube and then does not quite fill the blue-top tube.

Key Words: butterfly use • hemoconcentration • hemolysis • home health-care phlebotomy • inadequate electrolyte and prothrombin (PT) blood sample • nonadditive tubes • tissue thromboplastin contamination

QUESTIONS

1. Document and explain the errors Dave has committed.

2. Has Dave used the correct tubes and order of draw?

3. Are these blood samples usable? Why or why not?

DISCUSSION OF CASE STUDY

1. The phlebotomist has a very important role in the delivery of health care. Placing the patient at ease, obtaining an adequate blood sample, and ensuring that the blood sample is an accurate reflection of the patient's condition are the first steps in good health care. Dave is work-ing two jobs, was out late, and is too tired to exercise good judgment. He is probably grumpy and flustered from having to jump out of bed and rush to his first patient. He also did not have time to check whether he has all of the equipment and supplies he needs for his morning draws. He missed the vein in the antecubital area, and this indicates that he is not working at his optimum level.

    Because Mrs. P.S. is a very thin, elderly woman, it is likely her veins are fragile or sclerosed and tend to roll easily. She also needs a PT, which could indicate that she is taking a "blood thinner" and will there-fore bleed more easily. Dave needs to exercise good venipuncture tech-nique, such as holding the skin more tautly so the veins do not roll and applying additional pressure for a longer period of time once the venipuncture is complete (Fig. 4.6).

2. Veins in the hands tend to roll even more easily than in the antecubital area. Dave could have tried another vein in the antecubital area of Mrs. P.S.'s other arm. However, Dave decided to access the hand vein. The slow blood flow from the hand vein into the Vacutainer tube indicates that the butterfly needle is not centered well in the lumen of the vein or the vacuum pressure within the Vacutainer tube has partially collapsed the smaller, fragile hand veins of Mrs. P.S. (Fig. 4.7).

    Dave should have used smaller-volume Vacutainer tubes, which have less vacuum pressure, and of course used better technique in accessing the hand vein. The order of draw for the electrolyte panel and PT is **incorrect**. A plain (nonadditive) red-top or black-top tube should be

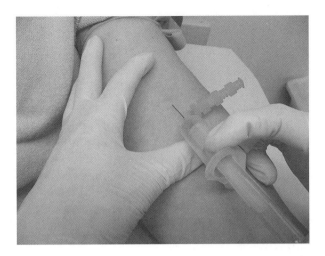

Figure 4.6. Technique for Holding a Vein in Place.

drawn before the blue-top tube to prevent tissue thromboplastin contamination and contamination by additives from other tubes. The green-top (lithium heparin) tube should be drawn last.

3. Neither of the blood specimens that were drawn is useable. Blood flowing very slowly into the green-top tube is likely to contribute to hemolysis. Dave probably has had to leave the tourniquet on longer than recommended, which will contribute to hemoconcentration of large molecules such as protein and cholesterol. Hemolysis of RBCs will result in release of additional potassium into the plasma. Even if no hemolysis is visible in the centrifuged blood specimen for the electrolytes, hemoconcentration will contribute to inaccurate results.

    An inadequate amount of blood in the blue-top tube will result in an abnormal proportion of anticoagulant and whole blood. The PT test is performed to assess clotting ability. If Mrs. P.S. is taking Coumadin or dicumarol, an accurate assessment of how well these drugs are suppressing her clotting ability is essential. An accurate test is impossible if the blue-top citrate blood specimen is inadequate.

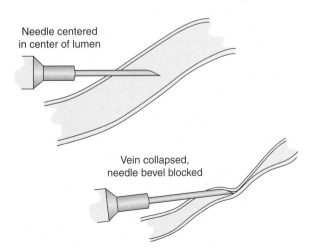

Needle centered
in center of lumen

Vein collapsed,
needle bevel blocked

Figure 4.7. Diagram of Collapsed Vein; Position of Needle.

CASE 27
Fasting and Family Members

Mrs. M.R. is an elderly Hispanic woman who speaks only Spanish and needs blood drawn for a fasting lipid. Anna is an experienced phlebotomist. She enters the patient's room and finds four family members with Mrs. M.R. They all begin talking at once, telling Anna she should draw the blood from Mrs. M.R.'s left arm. There are no signs above Mrs. M.R.'s bed indicating special treatment of either arm. Anna notices that there are numerous food items on Mrs. M.R.'s bedside table.

Key Words: cultural issues • fasting

QUESTIONS

1. What should Anna do?

2. Does it make a difference whether Anna speaks Spanish or not?

DISCUSSION OF CASE STUDY

1. In Hispanic culture, close family ties are very important. Anna needs to be cognizant of and to honor these ties; however, she must also create an environment comfortable for her and her patient. Anna needs to introduce herself and very diplomatically ask if the family will designate one person as their representative to remain with Mrs. M.R. while Anna does her job. There are two issues to consider here. One issue is whether there is a good reason for drawing from Mrs. M.R.'s left arm, and the other is for Anna to determine whether Mrs. M.R. is indeed fasting and has not had anything to eat recently. To determine the answers to these two questions, Anna will need to ask Mrs. M.R., the designated family representative, or the nurse in charge of Mrs. M.R.

2. It certainly would be easier to question the patient and the family members if Anna spoke Spanish. However, in establishing a family representative, Anna could ask if one of them speaks English and could act as an interpreter or perhaps ask one of the nurses to interpret for her. There may be a good reason for Anna to draw the blood from Mrs. M.R.'s left arm. A previous phlebotomist may have tried the other arm and failed or left a large bruise. Mrs. M.R. may have had a mastectomy on her right side. Mrs. M.R. may be a kidney dialysis patient and have an AV shunt in the right arm. With a careful examination of Mrs. M.R.'s right arm, Anna should be able to ascertain whether these are possible reasons. With the latter two possibilities, the nursing staff should have a sign posted indicating that the right arm should not be used (Fig. 4.8).

   The other question that must be answered is whether Mrs. M.R. is really fasting or not. A fasting blood sample requires that the patient has not eaten for approximately 12 hours before collection of the specimen.

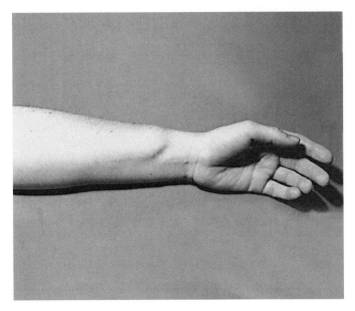

Figure 4.8. Internal AV Shunt (Fistula).

Mrs. M.R. can drink water, but nothing else by mouth. Anna needs to explain that if Mrs. M.R. has eaten anything recently, her blood test (fasting lipid) will be abnormal and it is not worthwhile to draw her blood at this time.

CASE 28
Hematoma Formation

Mrs. M.S. is a large, overweight, elderly woman who needs blood drawn for electrolytes, CBC, and a prothrombin time. Mimi is a new phlebotomist at the local blood drawing center who must collect the blood sample from Mrs. M.S. Mimi correctly verifies the identification of the patient by asking Mrs. M.S. her name and date of birth. Mimi then selects the tubes she needs, prepares the Vacutainer, and selects the optimal site for venipuncture. Mimi carefully palpates the antecubital area of Mrs. M.S.'s left arm and is only able to locate the cephalic vein. Because Mrs. M.S. has very large arms, Mimi can only feel a small portion of the vein, and she therefore enters the vein at a larger angle than normal. Blood slowly enters the Vacutainer tube. Mimi also notices that a raised area is forming around the needle. Mimi has only one more tube to collect and therefore fills the third tube before withdrawing the Vacutainer from the vein.

Key Words: cephalic vein • hematoma formation • hemolysis • obese patients • optimum needle angle • vessel lumen

QUESTIONS

1. What is the best choice of veins for venipuncture?
2. What is the normal angle for needle penetration of a vein?
3. Is the blood sample that Mimi obtained useful?
4. What tubes does Mimi need for the electrolytes, CBC, and prothrombin time? What is the order of draw?
5. What did Mimi do wrong?

DISCUSSION OF CASE STUDY

1. The best choice of veins for venipuncture is usually the median cubital vein. The best choice for patient arm, whether right or left, is usually the patient's dominant arm because the veins are larger. If Mrs. M.S. is right-handed, her right arm would have been a better choice. Mrs. M.S. is also overweight. The additional fatty tissue in the arm may prevent easy visualization of veins in the antecubital area. The cephalic vein is on the same side as the thumb, or an easy way to remember this vein is when the patient is in anatomic position (hands to the side, palmar side up), the cephalic vein is closest to the head. The cephalic vein is a second choice because it tends to roll more easily. However, this was the only vein Mimi was able to locate.

2. The normal angle for penetration of a vein is usually 15° to 30°. Mimi used a larger angle to access Mrs. M.S.'s vein. With a larger angle, it is more difficult to control the depth of penetration and to ensure that the beveled edge of the needle is really in the center of the vessel lumen. The lumen is the interior space within the vein. Mimi either has not fully entered the lumen of the vein or has gone through the lumen and partially penetrated the other side of the vein (Fig. 4.9). As a result, blood is leaking around the site(s) of needle penetration and into the surrounding tissues—a hematoma is forming.

3. With blood leakage into the surrounding tissue, hemolysis of blood cells and activation of clotting factors is likely to occur. The hemolysis will cause measurements of electrolytes to be inaccurate, particularly K^+. The number of RBCs in the CBC and therefore the hematocrit and hemoglobin determination will be decreased. Activation of clotting factors will result in an inaccurate prothrombin time. The blood sample will not be useful.

4. Mimi needs a green-top tube for the electrolytes, a lavender-top tube for the CBC, and a blue-top tube for the prothrombin time. If using a Vacutainer, usually a blue discard tube needs to be drawn before the prothrombin time. The blue prothrombin time tube is followed by the green-top tube for electrolytes. The lavender-top tube for the CBC is last.

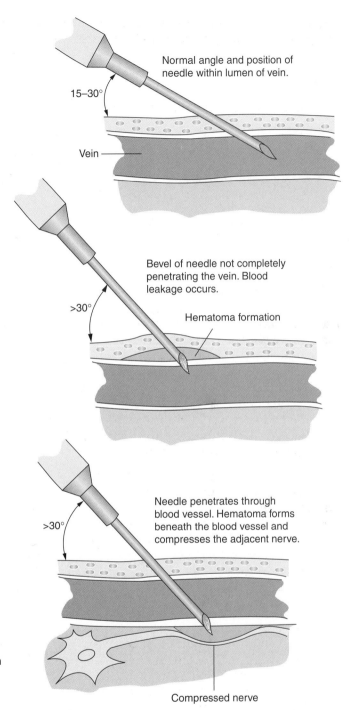

Normal angle and position of needle within lumen of vein.

15–30°

Vein

Bevel of needle not completely penetrating the vein. Blood leakage occurs.

>30°

Hematoma formation

Needle penetrates through blood vessel. Hematoma forms beneath the blood vessel and compresses the adjacent nerve.

>30°

Compressed nerve

Figure 4.9. Formation of Hematoma Due to Incorrect Needle Positioning.

5. Mimi used too large an angle for access to the vein, leading to the formation of a hematoma. As soon as she noticed that a hematoma was forming, she should have immediately withdrawn the needle and applied pressure to the site to stop any further subcutaneous bleeding. A hematoma can be dangerous because pressure from the blood accumulating blood at the site can damage surrounding nerves and result in temporary or permanent damage.

Quiz

MULTIPLE CHOICE

1. A well-known organization for accrediting hospitals is ____.
   a. JCAHO
   b. NACCLS
   c. NIH
   d. NCQA
   e. HCFA

2. To correctly identify a patient, the following can be used ___.
   a. patient complete name
   b. date of birth
   c. identification number of ID card
   d. a and b
   e. a, b, and c

3. The term geriatric refers to ___.
   a. joint disease
   b. elderly people
   c. rehabilitation facility
   d. senility
   e. loss of hearing

4. When working with the elderly, phlebotomists need to be aware of ___.
   a. physical disabilities
   b. emotional problems
   c. mental problems
   d. a and b
   e. a, b, and c

5. Common physical disabilities occurring in the elderly include ___.
   a. arthritis
   b. loss of hearing
   c. blindness
   d. a and b
   e. a, b, and c

6. Which of the following is an example of an electrolyte?
   a. Na$^+$
   b. Cl$^+$
   c. Fe
   d. a and b
   e. a, b, and c

7. Causes of dehydration include ___.
   a. vomiting
   b. profuse sweating
   c. decreased intake of fluids
   d. a and b
   e. a, b, and c

8. Which of the following substances has different normal levels in the blood at different times of the day?
   a. estrogen
   b. CK isoenzymes
   c. lactic acid
   d. serum iron
   e. alkaline phosphatase

9. Serum iron requires a ____ top tube.
   a. royal blue
   b. gold
   c. lavender
   d. green
   e. light blue

10. The patient needs electrolytes, a liver panel, CBC, and Fe drawn. If using a Vacutainer, which tube is drawn first?
    a. gold
    b. lavender
    c. green
    d. black
    e. yellow

11. Which of the following tests requires an ice slurry for transport of the blood sample?
    a. BUN
    b. creatinine
    c. liver panel
    d. ammonia
    e. erythrocyte sedimentation rate

12. Which of the following tests usually requires the patient to be fasting?
    a. lipids
    b. cholesterol
    c. triglycerides
    d. a and b
    e. a, b, and c

13. Fasting means that patient has not eaten for approximately ___ hours before the blood sample is drawn.
    a. 12
    b. 8
    c. 6
    d. 4
    e. 2

14. Valid reason(s) for *not* drawing a blood sample from one arm is/are ___.
    a. presence of a hematoma or bruise
    b. a mastectomy on that side
    c. presence of an AV shunt
    d. a and b
    e. a, b, and c

15. To verify if a patient is fasting ___.
    a. note if food items are nearby
    b. ask the nurse in charge
    c. ask the patient
    d. ask family members
    e. all of the above

16. Cultural sensitivity means ___.
    a. understanding customs of different peoples
    b. working with a patient's family
    c. being able to speak a foreign language
    d. asking all family members to leave a patient's room so you can do your job
    e. a and b

17. The best choice for drawing blood from the antecubital area is ___.
    a. cephalic vein
    b. basilica vein
    c. median cubital vein
    d. brachial vein
    e. ulnar vein

18. The normal angle for penetration of a vein is ____.
   a. 5° to 10°
   b. 15° to 30°
   c. 20° to 40°
   d. 30° to 45°

19. The vessel lumen is ___.
   a. interior diameter
   b. exterior diameter
   c. interior space
   d. wall of the blood vessel
   e. junction of veins

20. A raised area around a venipuncture site is a ____.
   a. bruise
   b. hematoma
   c. petechiae
   d. aneurysm
   e. hemarthrosis

21. Hemolysis in a blood sample will result in ___.
   a. loss of RBCs
   b. release of hemoglobin
   c. release of K^+
   d. a and b
   e. a, b, and c

22. Nerve damage may occur as a result of poor venipuncture technique because ___.
   a. nerve is penetrated by needle
   b. hematoma formation causes pressure against the nerve
   c. hemolysis is toxic to the nerve
   d. a and b
   e. a, b, and c

23. To determine which antibiotics are useful for treating a patient with a *Pseudomonas* infection, a(n) ___ test is performed.
   a. antibiotic peak
   b. antibiotic trough
   c. antibiotic sensitivity
   d. antibiotic resistance
   e. BUN

24. To measure when antibiotic levels are at a maximum, a ____ specimen must be drawn.
  a. trough
  b. peak
  c. toxicity
  d. base level
  e. therapeutic

MATCH THE ERROR IN BLOOD DRAWING WITH THE OUTCOME.

25. leaving tourniquet on too long   a. hematoma

26. penetrating through the vein   b. hemolysis

27. inadequate blood sample in   c. hemoconcentration
        sodium citrate tube
                                                d. prolonged clotting time

                                                e. a and b

ESSAY QUESTIONS

28. Describe tissue changes in elderly people that phlebotomists need to be aware of in drawing a blood sample.

29. Describe mental and emotional changes that occur in elderly people that phlebotomists need to be aware of to ensure optimum blood drawing conditions.

30. Explain how dehydration may affect blood test results.

31. Careful observation of the patient's behavior is especially necessary with an order for a blood ammonia test. Explain why. What precautions should be taken?

32. What precautions are necessary when accessing a hand vein? What if the patient is taking Coumadin?

33. Explain why it is important to accurately obtain a timed peak and trough blood sample.

CHAPTER 5

Ethical, Legal, and Regulatory Issues

CASE 29
Quality Assurance and Contaminated Blood Cultures

Meg draws a blood culture set from patient C.P. at 8 AM. The physician orders a blood culture while the patient is spiking a fever (11 AM). One of the nurses draws this blood culture set. Two days later, the microbiology department reports that both sets of blood cultures from patient C.P. were contaminated with ***Staphylococcus epidermidis*** (a normal skin flora bacteria). All contaminated blood cultures for each quarter of the year are reported to the Laboratory Quality Assurance (QA) Committee. The report contains information concerning how many contaminated blood cultures occurred during the previous 3-month time period and who obtained the blood cultures. Meg is found to have a higher rate of contaminated blood cultures than the other phlebotomists. Nursing has an even higher rate of contamination (8%). NCCLS recommends that a contamination rate of <5% is acceptable.

Key Words: chlorhexidine and alcohol • contaminated blood cultures
• correct procedures for obtaining blood cultures • NCCLS
• Quality Assurance (QA) • Quality Control (QC)
• sodium polyanethol sulfonate (SPS)

QUESTIONS

1. What does a contaminated blood culture mean to the patient?
2. What is the correct procedure for obtaining a blood culture?
3. What can be done to resolve the problem with Meg?
4. What can be done to resolve the contamination rate of blood cultures by nurses?
5. What is Quality Assurance?
6. What does NCCLS stand for? Who is NCCLS?

DISCUSSION OF CASE STUDY

1. The physician ordered the blood culture because she suspects that the patient may have bacteremia, a serious condition in which bacteria are circulating and causing an infection in the blood. A positive blood culture confirms that the patient does have bacteremia, and from the bacterial growth in the blood culture medium, the organism causing the infection can be isolated, identified, and tested for antibiotic susceptibility. Antibiotic susceptibility indicates which antibiotics are most effective at controlling growth of the bacteria, and because many pathogenic bacteria are becoming antibiotic resistant, it is important to identify which antibiotic will work best against this bug. If the blood culture is contaminated with normal flora bacteria such as *Staph. epidermidis*, it is impossible to confirm that the patient has bacteremia. Avoiding contamination is essential.

2. Correct procedures for obtaining a blood culture are designed to ensure that contamination is minimized. Meg should briefly explain the test to the patient. She should then ask the patient if he or she is allergic to latex or iodine. If the patient is allergic to iodine, alcohol may be used in place of iodine (Figs. 5.1 and 5.2).

   After donning gloves and locating the vein to be used, the tourniquet is loosened and the venipuncture site is cleaned carefully with a sterile alcohol pad. Start in the center of the area to be cleansed, and with a circular motion work outward. Rub with moderate pressure. It is important to use some pressure to help the alcohol penetrate and cleanse the deeper layers of skin.

   This is followed by a second cleansing with iodine; apply iodine to the cleansed area. Start the application again in the center of the cleansed area and work outward. Movement of the iodine tincture should be in outward circles, covering an area approximately 4 inches in diameter. No overlap in concentric circles should occur. Allow the iodine to dry (30 to 60 seconds). Iodine and alcohol are being replaced

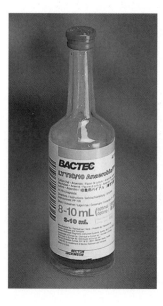

Figure 5.1.   Bactec Blood Culture Bottle.

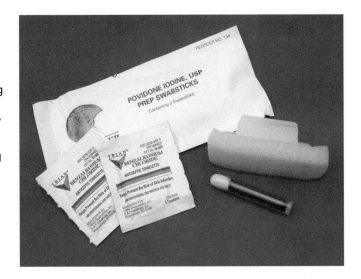

Figure 5.2. Three Types of Blood Culture Cleaning Supplies. Left, Povidone-Iodine Swabsticks. Center, Benzalkonium Chloride. Right, Frepp/Sepp Povidone-Iodine Cleaning Kit Components. (Reprinted with Permission from McCall RE, Tankersley CM. Phlebotomy Essentials. 3rd Ed. Philadelphia: Lippincott Williams & Wilkins, 2003.)

at many hospitals with chlorhexidine and alcohol solutions that require only one application.

Meg should use the drying time to prepare the blood culture vials. Swab the rubber stopper of the blood culture bottles with an alcohol wipe. Leave the alcohol wipe on the rubber stopper for 1 minute. Remove the alcohol wipe and allow the rubber stopper to dry. DO NOT TOUCH THE STERILE RUBBER STOPPERS. Historically, iodine was used on the rubber stoppers before swabbing with the alcohol pad. Iodine was eliminated because the rubber stoppers deteriorated from the iodine.

Meg should now retie the tourniquet. Once the arm has been cleaned and prepared, Meg cannot place her finger on the spot to be punctured. If necessary, Meg can clean her gloved finger with alcohol or chlorhexidine for relocating the vein.

The blood can be drawn into a safety syringe, and, using a sterile transfer device, is delivered first into the anaerobic vial and then the aerobic. The blood can also be drawn using a butterfly and a direct-draw adaptor that fits the blood culture vial. All materials must be handled aseptically. With a butterfly, the blood is delivered into the aerobic vial first because the tubing will contain air. The anaerobic vial is then filled. A third method for drawing a blood culture uses culture vials designed to fit safety-holder needle apparatuses or yellow-topped evacuated tubes containing sodium polyanethol sulfonate (SPS). The tops of these tubes and vials are not sterile and need to be wiped with iodine and alcohol. Sodium polyanethol sulfonate is an additive that will prevent coagulation by binding to calcium. It will also enhance the growth of bacteria because it inhibits complement and phagocytosis and reduces the activity of certain antibiotics.

If other blood tests are also ordered, the blood culture is drawn *first* to avoid contamination by other tubes. Blood cultures cannot be obtained through intravenous catheters because these indwelling lines become contaminated with bacteria themselves.

3. Meg needs to review correct blood culture drawing procedures to identify where she may be inadvertently introducing contamination.

She and the phlebotomy supervisor also need to discuss and review exactly what Meg is doing to contribute to her higher contamination rate and determine ways she can improve.

4. A workshop for the nurses could be organized to review correct procedures and ways to improve their contamination rate. Alternatively, blood could be drawn exclusively by the phlebotomists. This might entail more coordination and communication between the nursing staff and laboratory so that phlebotomists are more readily available when patients are spiking a fever.

5. QA or continuous quality improvement (CQI) are procedures or processes developed to improve health care. Quality health care is a concept that involves all health care personnel, patients, hospital administration, the community, government, accrediting agencies, physical facilities, etc. The health care services that are provided to patients must be appropriate and performed in a manner that will benefit the patient. In the case of improving blood culture contamination rates, QA procedures need to be developed with the cooperation and communication of appropriate laboratory supervisors, phlebotomists, and nursing staff to ensure optimum outcomes and benefits for patients.

  QA differs from quality control (QC) in that QC is concerned with the accuracy of individual tests and the performance of calibration controls, checking instrumentation, temperature, and other variables of the test itself.

6. The National Committee for Clinical Laboratory Standards (NCCLS) is a national nonprofit organization composed of representatives from clinical laboratories, industry, and government that develops guidelines and standards for all functions of the clinical laboratory, including recommended blood culture contamination rates and optimal procedures, materials, and reagents for obtaining and analyzing blood cultures.

CASE 30
Lab Safety/Fire

A small fire occurred in a white-bagged trash can. Pat, the phlebotomist, immediately grabbed the B-type fire extinguisher and swept over the top of the fire. The fire expanded to the surrounding area.

Key Words: classes of fire • NFPA • PASS • RACE • types of fire extinguishers

QUESTIONS

1. What did Pat do wrong?

2. What does the acronym PASS refer to? Explain.

3. What does the acronym RACE refer to? Explain.

4. What needs to be done next?

DISCUSSION OF CASE STUDY

1. The National Fire Protection Agency (NFPA) identifies four classes of fires: Class A, B, C, and D. Class A fires occur with ordinary combustible material such as wood, paper, or clothing. Class B fires involve flammable liquids and vapors such as paint, oil, grease, or gasoline. Class C fires involve electrical equipment, and Class D fires occur with combustible or reactive metals such as sodium potassium, magnesium, or lithium.

    Pat grabbed a B-type fire extinguisher that is for flammable liquids. The white-bagged trash can is for paper goods, and therefore is a Class A type fire. Class A type fire extinguishers contain soda and acid or water and are used to cool the fire. Class B extinguishers contain foam, dry chemicals, or carbon dioxide to smother the fire. Class C fire extinguishers have similar ingredients and likewise smother a fire. Pat should have grabbed the A-type fire extinguisher or a multipurpose class ABC extinguisher to take care of the initially simple fire in the trash can.

2. The acronym PASS stands for *P*ull the pin, *A*im the nozzle, *S*queeze the trigger, and *S*weep the nozzle (Fig. 5.3). Pat may have remembered this acronym; however, she still used the extinguisher incorrectly. She should have swept the **base** of the fire. Sweeping over the top can spread the fire further. And, of course, she used the wrong fire extinguisher.

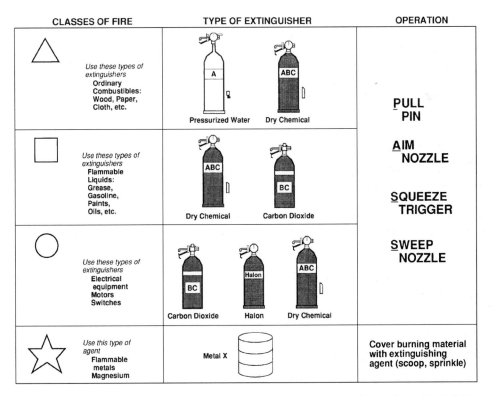

Figure 5.3. Classes of Fire Extinguishers. (Reprinted with Permission from McCall RE, Tankersley CM. Phlebotomy Essentials. 3rd Ed. Philadelphia: Lippincott Williams & Wilkins, 2003.)

3. Because Pat did not use the correct fire extinguisher and the fire is spreading, Pat now needs to use the acronym RACE. The R refers to rescue of any individuals in danger, A stands for sound the alarm, C stands for confine the fire by closing all doors and windows, and E stands for extinguish the fire with the nearest appropriate fire extinguisher.

4. Pat needs to make sure she does not panic and run. She should call for help, and hopefully there is an appropriate fire extinguisher handy so that this fire does not get any larger. Pat needs to review fire safety procedures, and make sure she knows the difference between the classes of fires and types of fire extinguishers so that a similar incident does not occur again.

CASE 31
Liability/Scope of Practice

Jenny has recently completed her phlebotomy training and obtained her certification. She has an order for a liver panel and CBC for Mrs. M.S. Mrs. M.S. is a very large woman who is in the hospital because she recently had surgery for removal of her gallbladder. Using a Vacutainer, Jenny draws a lavender-top tube and then a gold-top tube. However, before Jenny is able to leave the room, the patient asks for help to get to the bathroom. Jenny attempts to help Mrs. M.S., but on the way to the bathroom, the patient falls and fractures her arm.

Key Words: "deeper pockets" • defendant • independent contractor • liability • plaintiff • scope of practice • vicarious liability

QUESTIONS

1. Should Jenny have tried to help the patient to the restroom? Is she liable for the patient's injury?

2. If there was water left on the floor, does this change who is liable? Explain.

3. If Jenny works for a laboratory that contracts with the hospital to provide blood drawing and testing, does this change the liability? Explain.

4. Did Jenny draw the correct tubes and in the correct order?

DISCUSSION OF CASE STUDY

1. Jenny should *not* have helped the patient to the bathroom. Patient assistance in this capacity is *not* within her scope of practice. Scope of practice is the standard of care that should be rendered by a phlebotomist. Jenny has not been trained in assessing whether this patient is ready to walk to the bathroom, nor is she trained in the correct procedures for aiding a patient to be mobile after surgery. She is liable for the patient's injury. The patient could file a lawsuit against Jenny. In legal terms,

Mrs. M.S. would then be the plaintiff and Jenny would be the defendant. Jenny should have told Mrs. M.S. that although she could not help Mrs. M.S. to the bathroom, she would alert one of the nurses at the nurses' station that Mrs. M.S. needs to use the bathroom.

2. Not only is Jenny liable, but because of the "deeper pockets" doctrine, Mrs. M.S. can also sue the hospital and independent contractor that Jenny works for. The deeper pockets doctrine allows the plaintiff to collect from the codefendants with the most money. If there were water left on the floor, this fact would probably shift more of the liability burden onto the hospital because their cleaning personnel did not immediately mop the water spill. However, Jenny is still liable because she should not have helped Mrs. M.S. get out of bed in the first place.

3. Current health care delivery services more frequently include independent contractors. A company can be formed to provide certain services. The company then forms a contract with the hospital. This company hires employees, pays these employees, and bills the hospital for services rendered. The radiology department may be an independent contractor. The radiologist can rent space from the hospital, and can then hire x-ray technicians and other necessary personnel, pay their salaries, even bill patients separately from the hospital.

   In Jenny's case, she works for a phlebotomy company. This company hires phlebotomists, pays their salaries, and probably bills the hospital for the phlebotomists' time and skills. Hopefully, they also maintain liability insurance. However, the hospital can still be held responsible as well because of vicarious liability. The hospital hires the independent contractor and is therefore responsible for ensuring that the independent contractor and their employees are fully trained and can deliver the standard of care necessary for phlebotomy (See Box 5.1).

BOX 5.1

GUIDELINES FOR AVOIDING LAWSUITS

- Acquire informed consent before collection of specimens.
- Respect a patient's right to confidentiality.
- Strictly adhere to accepted procedures and practices.
- Use proper safety containers and devices.
- Listen and respond appropriately to the patient's requests.
- Accurately and legibly record all information concerning patients.
- Document incidents or occurrences.
- Participate in continuing education to maintain proficiency.
- Perform at the prevailing standard of care.
- Never perform procedures that you are not trained to do.

Reprinted with permission from McCall RE, Tankersley CM. Phlebotomy Essentials. 3rd Ed. Philadelphia: Lippincott Williams & Wilkins, 2003.

4. Jenny drew the correct tubes: lavender-top tube with EDTA as the anticoagulant of choice for CBCs and gold-top tube containing a clot activator and gel separator for the liver panel tests. However, she did *not* draw the tubes in the correct order. A lavender-top tube is drawn last because of the possibility of carry-over of EDTA to the gold-top tube. The gold-top tube is designed for serum formation. See Table 5.1 for a detailed listing of tubes and the correct order. If EDTA contaminates the gold-top tube, clotting may not occur efficiently and test results may be compromised (see Table 5.1).

CASE 32
Responsible Behavior

Juan is a home health care phlebotomist who has a requisition for Mr. J.S., an elderly gentleman on three-times-per-week kidney dialysis. Mr. J.S. has an AV shunt in his left arm. Juan is able to draw blood for an electrolyte panel, BUN, creatinine, and CBC from his other arm. He places the tubes in a biohazard bag and quickly leaves. Because this is Juan's last pick-up for the day, he makes a quick stop at the bank. However, there is a long line and Juan ends up spending 45 minutes in the bank. It takes 2 hours to get back to the laboratory because of heavy traffic. Mr. J.S.'s blood samples sit another hour in the laboratory before tests are run.

Key Words: arteriovenous shunt • dialysis • electrolytes • fistula • glycolysis

QUESTIONS

1. What tubes are needed for drawing these tests? What anticoagulants are necessary? Would sodium heparin be a good choice and why?

2. Are any of the tests time sensitive?

3. Why should the arm with the AV shunt be avoided for blood drawing?

4. Did Juan behave responsibly? How can Juan be held accountable?

DISCUSSION OF CASE STUDY

1. An electrolyte panel includes sodium (Na^+), potassium (K^+) and chloride (Cl^-). The kidney has a major role in assuring normal levels of these important ions in the blood. Mr. J.S. has evidently suffered some type of kidney disease and has limited or no kidney function. Therefore he must undergo kidney dialysis. The dialysis process will help maintain normal levels of electrolytes. Likewise, blood urea nitrogen levels (BUN) and creatinine are metabolic waste products that the kidney normally eliminates. These blood components must be carefully monitored.

TABLE 5.1

NCCLS Order of Draw, Stopper Color, and Rationale for Collection Order

Order of Draw	Tube Stopper Color	Rationale for Collection Order
Blood cultures (sterile collections)	Yellow sodium polyanetholsulfonate (SPS) (or sterile media containers)	Minimizes chance of microbial contamination
Plain (nonadditive) tubes	Red	Prevents contamination by additives in other tubes
Coagulation tubes	Light blue	Second or third position in order of draw prevents tissue thromboplastin contamination
		Must be the first additive tube in the order because all other additive tubes affect coagulation tests
Serum separator gel tubes (SSTs)	Red and gray rubber Gold plastic	Prevents contamination by additives in other tubes. Comes after coagulation tests because silica particles activate clotting and affect coagulation tests; carryover of silica into subsequent tubes can be overridden by the anticoagulant in them
Plasma separator gel tubes (PSTs)	Green and gray rubber Light green plastic	Contains heparin, which affects coagulation tests and interferes in collection of serum specimens; causes the least interference in tests other than coagulation tests
Heparin tubes	Green	Same as PST
Ethylenediaminetetraacetic acid (EDTA) tubes	Lavender	Causes more carryover problems than any other additive; elevates sodium and potassium levels; chelates and decreases calcium and iron levels; elevates prothrombin time and partial thromboplastin time results
Oxalate/fluoride tubes	Gray	Sodium fluoride and potassium oxalate elevate sodium and potassium levels, respectively; comes after hematology tubes because oxalate damages cell membranes and causes abnormal red blood cell morphology

Reprinted with permission from McCall RE, Tankersley CM. Phlebotomy Essentials. 3rd Ed. Philadelphia: Lippincott Williams & Wilkins, 2003.

The blood sample for the electrolyte panel, BUN, and creatinine should be drawn into a green-top lithium heparin tube, **not** a sodium heparin tube. The sodium heparin will contaminate the blood sample and yield a falsely high sodium level. The CBC is drawn into a lavender-top tube that contains EDTA.

2. The electrolytes are time-sensitive. The plasma cannot remain in contact with the RBCs for more than 2 to 4 hours. The plasma must be separated within 2 to 4 hours. If the plasma is not separated, the potassium level will increase because of glycolysis and leakage from the RBCs. Glucose will also decrease because of glycolysis. RBCs are still alive in the tubes, which means they continue to use glucose and release potassium as a by-product. The cells in the CBC tube will begin to change at approximately 8 hours.

3. AV refers to an arteriovenous shunt or a fistula. An artery and a vein are surgically connected to allow easy access for kidney dialysis. The connection is usually close to the surface of the skin and can be seen and felt (see Fig. 4.8).

   A tourniquet or blood pressure cuff should never be used on an arm with a shunt because damage could occur to this important vascular access procedure. Nor should blood be drawn from this arm. A nurse specially trained in kidney dialysis procedures may provide a blood sample from an AV shunt portal for testing. This blood sample should be labeled regarding its source because test results may be different from blood obtained from a normal vein.

4. Juan did **not** behave responsibly. Even though this was his last pick-up for the day, he is still on the job. It is his responsibility not only to draw the blood specimen, but also to deliver that specimen back to the laboratory in a timely manner to ensure accurate test results. Mr. J.S.'s blood samples were not tested until almost 4 hours after being drawn. Even if Juan had the samples in a refrigerated or cooled container, the electrolyte results might still be abnormally high. Hopefully, the abnormally high electrolyte results would be questioned by the technologist/CLS and the physician. If Mr. J.S.'s physician were to accept the results as being accurate, the physician likely would recommend lengthening dialysis time, which could be very dangerous to Mr. J.S.

   In most laboratories, the abnormal test results can be traced back to the phlebotomist who drew the blood sample. If Juan is an ethically responsible person, he would alert his supervisor that the samples he delivered for Mr. J.S. remained in his car for an abnormally long period of time and that this incident would not occur again.

CASE 33
Combative Patient

Jeanine is the phlebotomist called into the blood drawing room to draw a lithium and testosterone level from D.P. D.P. is a 17-year-old white male patient with a developmental disability and a diagnosed mental age of

12. D.P. does not want to have his blood drawn and is combative. His uncles, who have accompanied him to the hospital, are willing to restrain D.P. while Jeanine draws his blood.

Key Words: incompetent patient • legal guardianship • lithium as a drug • minor • parental consent • testosterone

QUESTIONS

    1. What should Jeanine do?

    2. If the patient were age 23, would Jeanine's actions change?

    3. What tubes and anticoagulants are required for these tests?

DISCUSSION OF CASE STUDY

    1. This particular case involves many legal issues. At 17 years of age, D.P. is still considered a minor, at least in California and in many other states where the legal age of adults is considered to be 18. As a minor, **parental consent** for any type of medical treatment or procedure is required. The uncles of D.P. do not have authority to give consent unless they have been given legal guardianship.

    2. Because D.P. is mentally challenged, even if he were 23 he would be considered an incompetent patient; parental, guardian, or conservator consent still would be necessary before proceeding with blood drawing. Even if the uncles were legal guardians and were willing to restrain D.P., Jeanine should not risk drawing the blood sample. Phlebotomy is an invasive procedure. Injury to the patient and to Jeanine is a real possibility. D.P. might move, and if Jeanine missed the vein, she could be injured by an accidental needle stick. The blood tests ordered include lithium and testosterone levels. The patient is likely to be taking medication prescribed by his physician. Lithium is a drug used to treat psychiatric bipolar disorders. Jeanine should consult with her supervisor. The supervisor could then consult with the physician regarding how he or she would like to proceed with this patient.

    3. A blood specimen for lithium levels should be drawn into a green-top sodium heparin tube, *not* a lithium heparin tube. A 4-mL tube is an ample specimen. Testosterone is a sex hormone. The blood sample should be drawn into a SST tube. A 4-mL tube is ample. Plasma is also acceptable, either EDTA or heparin. The specimen should be centrifuged as soon as possible and the serum or plasma separated from the cells and frozen.

CASE 34
Interpersonal Communication Skills

Jane is a newly trained phlebotomist and has a requisition to draw a CBC from Mrs. M.Z. Mrs. M.Z. is in contact isolation because she has been diagnosed with an MRSA. Jane puts on a gown and enters the room with her tray. She turns on the light without announcing herself and discovers that Mrs. M.Z. is a frail, elderly Chinese woman who does not speak English. Jane attempts to explain that she is there to obtain a blood sample. She checks the patient's ID bracelet and pulls Mrs. M.Z.'s arm down. Mrs. M.Z. has arthritic hands and jerks her arm back. Jane tries again to force her arm down, but the patient resists. Mrs. M.Z.'s daughter is sitting in a nearby chair.

Key Words: arthritis • contact isolation • cultural issues • MRSA

QUESTIONS

1. What is an MRSA? Why is Mrs. M.Z. in contact isolation? What precautions need to be observed?

2. What errors has Jane committed?

3. How should Jane have handled the above situation?

4. What can Jane do to improve her interpersonal and communicative skills?

DISCUSSION OF CASE STUDY

1. MRSA stands for methicillin-resistant *Staphylococcus aureus*. This is a particularly dangerous strain of *Staph. aureus*. It is completely resistant to commonly prescribed penicillin-type antibiotics.

   Mrs. M.Z. is most likely in a private room designated for contact isolation because she has an MRSA infection. It is imperative that standard precautions and contact precautions be observed so that this dangerous antibiotic-resistant bacteria is not spread to other patients. To ensure that this bacterial infection is not spread, Jane should wear gloves when entering the room, remove her gloves after completing procedures, and wash her hands immediately thereafter. She should wear a gown when entering the room and remove the gown before leaving. Only the blood drawing equipment needed should be taken into the room, and other materials and equipment should be left outside or at the nurses' station. Jane should review isolation procedures used by her work place.

2. Just because isolation procedures must be observed does not mean good communication skills are also left outside the door. Jane must still establish good rapport with the patient.

   Even though Mrs. M.Z. does not speak English, she may understand some English and certainly understands common courtesy. Jane did not knock on the door and announce herself before entering and turning on the light. Nor did she acknowledge Mrs. M.Z.'s daughter. Jane did not observe Mrs. M.Z.'s arthritic condition, and did not treat her very gently.

   Arthritis can be very painful and is fairly common in elderly women. A patient with arthritis can be identified by observing the hands. There are two forms of arthritis: osteoarthritis (OA) and rheumatoid arthritis (RA).

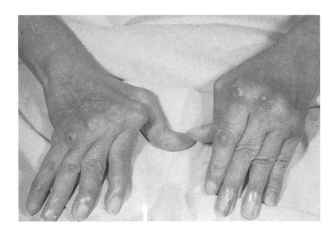

Figure 5.4. Arthritic Hands. (Reprinted with Permission from Rubin E, Farber JL. Pathology. 3rd Ed. Philadelphia: Lippincott Williams & Wilkins, 2000.)

OA is a result of wear and tear with age. RA is an autoimmune disease that has a three times higher frequency in women than in men. In both types of arthritis, joint inflammation occurs and bony overgrowths and misshapen joints of the hands are often seen. RA is usually much more aggressive and serious. The disease is debilitating and painful. With progression of the disease, more joints are involved and the patient becomes more disabled. In the case of Mrs. M.Z., she may also have arthritis in her elbow and shoulder and cannot readily straighten her arm without pain (Fig. 5.4).

3. The better approach for Jane would have been to knock and announce herself at the door, and explain who she is and her purpose for entering the room. She should have forewarned Mrs. M.Z. that she needed to turn on the light. At this point Jane should have noticed Mrs. M.Z.'s daughter sitting nearby and greeted her as well.

   Patients must consent to have a blood sample drawn. Consent may take the form of an actual written or verbal agreement or an implied consent in which the patient remains silent and cooperative. The patient has the right to know that the phlebotomist is part of the hospital staff and that the physician has ordered tests that require drawing a blood sample.

   Mrs. M.Z. jerked her arm back when Jane attempted to prepare Mrs. M.Z. for venipuncture. Mrs. M.Z. probably did not understand why Jane was there. She may have experienced pain because of Jane's rough handling. Because Mrs. M.Z.'s daughter was sitting nearby, Jane could have elicited help in translating and maybe in assisting to help hold Mrs. M.Z.'s arm. A family member can be very helpful in reassuring the patient and providing a source of comfort and safety (Fig. 5.5).

4. Jane needs to work with her supervisor. Her supervisor can probably provide reading materials, workshops, and mentoring so that Jane can become more sensitive to patient needs. Jane needs to improve her verbal communication skills and to show respect, especially in Asian cultures, in which respect for elders is stressed. Jane needs to know when it is appropriate to include family members.

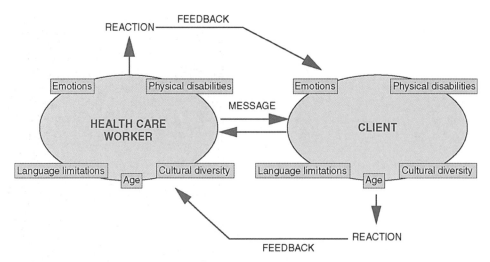

Figure 5.5. Communication Diagram. (Reprinted with Permission from McCall RE, Tankersley CM. Phlebotomy Essentials. 3rd Ed. Philadelphia: Lippincott Williams & Wilkins, 2003.)

CASE 35
Patient Identity and Ethics in the Workplace

Michelle has two patients with very similar names on her phlebotomy requisition list: Mrs. Elizabeth B. Brown and Mrs. Elizabeth M. Brown. When Michelle entered the room designated for Mrs. Elizabeth B. Brown, she found patient Elizabeth M., at least as indicated by the patient's ID bracelet. Michelle immediately reported the mix-up in patient location to the nurse's station. Mrs. Manley was at the desk and was the nurse in charge of these patients. Mrs. Manley was a good friend of Michelle's. When Michelle told Mrs. Manley of the mix-up in ID or location, Ms. Manley told her not to worry, she would fix the problem and because no harm had occurred, she did not think there was any need to report this problem to any other nurses or her supervisor.

Key Words: ethical behavior • importance of patient identification • incident report

QUESTIONS

1. What should Michelle do?

2. What problems may have occurred if Michelle had not noticed this error?

3. What ethical issues are present?

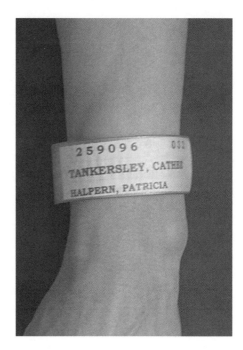

Figure 5.6. Identification Bracelet. (Reprinted with Permission from McCall RE, Tankersley CM. Phlebotomy Essentials. 3rd Ed. Philadelphia: Lippincott Williams & Wilkins, 2003.)

DISCUSSION OF CASE STUDY

1. Michelle acted correctly in carefully checking the patient's ID bracelet and immediately notifying the nurse's station of the mix-up in patient identification or location. Is the name on the patient's bracelet correct and is she in the wrong room, or vice versa? This is what needs to be determined immediately before other personnel become involved and before other procedures are erroneously performed on the wrong patient. Once verification of the patient identification and correct location is determined, Michele can then proceed with drawing the blood sample from the correct patient (Fig. 5.6).

2. Establishing the correct identification of a patient is imperative to avoid potential injury and even death. Based on test results belonging to the wrong patient, erroneous medication, blood transfusions, etc., may be given that could be life threatening. More errors of patient identification than technical errors contribute to transfusion reactions. Giving the wrong type of blood to a patient can be fatal. Legal consequences include malpractice suits and huge financial penalties for the personnel involved.

3. The ethical issue involved is Mrs. Manley's desire to *not* report this problem to a supervisor. Even though Michelle is a good friend, this incident should not be covered up. This is a serious problem that needs to be dealt with immediately so that further errors do not occur. A supervisor must be notified and this incident documented. Pertinent staff need to be alerted, and whoever was in error in initially establishing patient ID or location needs to realize the seriousness of the error. If Mrs. Manley does not notify a nursing supervisor, Michelle should certainly notify her phlebotomy supervisor and provide a written incident report.

CASE 36
Hematoma and Tingling Fingers

Mrs. K.F., a 48-year-old overweight woman, came to the outpatient blood-drawing center with a doctor's order for a PT. Madeline was the phlebotomist on duty at the time. Mrs. K.F. told Madeline that she had suffered a mild heart attack 2 months ago and is now on Coumadin. Madeline had difficulty finding a readily accessible vein and finally drew from the basilic vein at an approximately 35° angle. Madeline was able to obtain the blood sample. She withdrew the needle and had the patient apply pressure to the gauze pad. After labeling the tube, Madeline checked for any bleeding and sent the patient home. Later that day the patient called to report a large bruise and bump at the site of the blood draw and tingling of her fingers.

Key Words: basilic vein • hematoma • median nerve • nerve damage

QUESTIONS

1. What complications have occurred?
2. What is the recommended needle angle for entering a vein?
3. How severe is the problem?
4. Is Madeline liable for the injury to Mrs. K.F?
5. What corrective actions need to be taken?

DISCUSSION OF CASE STUDY

1. The veins in the antecubital fossa of a large, overweight woman such as Mrs. K.F. may be difficult to visualize and palpate. The vein of first choice for venipuncture is the median cubital because it is large and usually well anchored. However, the muscle and fat structure and exact locations of veins may differ slightly for every individual.

2. The ideal angle for inserting the needle into a vein is approximately a 15° angle with the needle following the lumen of the vein.

3. Madeline could not locate the median cubital vein or the cephalic vein of Mrs. K.F. and decided to attempt the basilic. The basilic is the last choice of appropriate veins in the antecubital fossa for venipuncture. This vein tends to roll, and the median nerve is located in close proximity. Madeline was able to enter the basilic vein at a 30° angle, which is *not* a good angle; it is too high and too acute. In the process of entering the vein at this angle she likely may have nicked or pierced through the other side. Furthermore, Mrs. K.F. is taking Coumadin, a medication that inhibits blood clotting. Additional pressure for 5 minutes or until bleeding has stopped is required for a normal blood draw on a patient taking anticoagulants. Even if Mrs. K.F. had not told Madeline she was taking Coumadin, the order for a PT should have alerted Madeline that she needed to apply pressure for a much longer time period.

BOX 5.2

SITUATIONS THAT MAY TRIGGER HEMATOMA FORMATION

1. The vein is fragile or too small for the needle size.

2. The needle penetrates all the way through the vein.

3. The needle is only partly inserted into the vein.

4. Excessive or blind probing is used to locate the vein.

5. The needle is removed while the tourniquet is still on.

6. Pressure is not adequately applied after venipuncture.

Reprinted with permission from McCall RE, Tankersley CM. Phlebotomy Essentials. 3rd Ed. Philadelphia: Lippincott Williams & Wilkins, 2003.

---

4. This is a severe problem because nerve damage is likely. The median nerve is a combined motor and sensory nerve. That means muscle movement and "feeling" in the fingers is controlled by this nerve. Tingling in the fingers indicates possible damage to the nerve. A hematoma has formed around the basilic vein, as indicated by the bruising and bump at the site where Madeline drew Mrs. K.F.'s blood (Box 5.2). The subcutaneous accumulation of blood at the site is pressing on the median nerve. Permanent damage to the nerve can occur. Madeline is liable for the injury to Mrs. K.F. She did not exercise good judgment in obtaining the blood sample, which includes the poor choice of a vein, too acute an angle for needle insertion, and failure to provide pressure for a long enough time after withdrawing the needle. Madeline, the blood-drawing center, the hospital, or the clinic could be sued for malpractice.

5. Madeline needs to immediately write an incident report to document exactly what happened and submit this to her supervisor. In case of a lawsuit, this report will be helpful in defending Madeline as the defendant, and in helping to recall the details of the incident that resulted in pain and suffering to the patient (the plaintiff). Lawsuits can be very costly. Malpractice insurance is available for individual health care workers. Most hospitals and clinical laboratories will also have malpractice insurance to cover their employees, including laboratory personnel. However, Madeline could lose her job and the least of the consequences she might suffer is that she needs some review and retraining to ensure that she is a competent phlebotomist with good judgment and skills.

CASE 37
Patient Dementia and Phlebotomist Negligence

Mrs. P.D. is 78-year-old white woman with dementia who needs blood drawn for an electrolyte panel and CBC. Louise, the phlebotomist, explains what she needs to do, and although the patient does not respond, she seems cooperative. Louise prepares her tubes and a Vacutainer holder with a needle, and then after examining Mrs. P.D.'s veins, realizes she needs to use a butterfly. Blood is obtained successfully, and Louise places a bandage on Mrs. P.D.'s arm and exits the room. Louise has inadvertently left the Vacutainer needle and holder on the bed. Mrs. P.D. finds the needle, removes the cap and attempts to sew her nightgown. Twenty minutes later, the nurse enters the patient's room and finds blood all over Mrs. P.D.'s nightgown and bedding from her pricked fingers.

Key Words: grounds for dismissal • legal issues • negligence • quality assurance

QUESTIONS

1. What is the outcome of this error? What is the outcome of the nursing response?

2. What is the effect on the patient?

3. What is the effect on the phlebotomist?

4. What are the legal and quality assurance issues?

5. What might the outcome be if the phlebotomist previously had been negligent?

DISCUSSION OF CASE STUDY

1. This is definitely a case of negligence, and fortunately Mrs. P.D. was not injured too badly. With serious injury, Louise or the laboratory could be sued for malpractice. The nursing staff needs to write an incident report that would be placed in Louise's employment file.

2. Mrs. P.D. will now need to have her fingers bandaged. Hopefully she does not have any other medical condition that will interfere with the healing process. Otherwise this incident could be complicated with infection.

3. The phlebotomy supervisor will need to speak to Louise, review correct procedures, and inform Louise that a report of this incident has been placed into her employment file. Also during their conversation, it should be determined whether there were circumstances that led to Louise's carelessness. Did she get enough sleep the night before? Were there some other personal or work-related issues that were distracting Louise? Having identified possible causes that may have led Louise to forget to clear the patient's bedside, corrective actions can be taken so that this incident is not repeated.

4. This incident will also reflect badly on the hospital. Mrs. P.D.'s relatives may come to visit. They will notice the bandages on Mrs. P.D.'s fingers and will want to know what happened. They will want to know who

was responsible and what kind of measures will be taken to ensure that this kind of negligence does not occur again.

5. If Louise has a history of negligence, this incident could lead to dismissal.

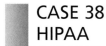

CASE 38
HIPAA

Susan, a phlebotomist, entered Miss Jones's room to draw some blood. Miss Jones was in the hospital for short-stay surgery, a therapeutic abortion. Miss Jones's physician had ordered a CBC, Lytes, PT, PTT, ABO/Rh, and Rhogam if indicated. While Susan was drawing the blood, Miss Jones's father was looking at the physician's orders.

Mr. Jones asked Susan what kind of test Rhogam is and what is meant by ... "if indicated"...? Susan told Mr. Jones that when an Rh-negative mother has an Rh-positive baby, the mom is given Rhogam to prevent the formation of antibodies against future pregnancies of Rh-positive babies.

Susan immediately noticed that the father and the daughter were visibly upset. The father said that the orders were wrong and that Susan should check with her supervisor. His daughter was not pregnant; she was having a simple corrective surgery.

Key Words: HIPAA • patient confidentiality • physician's orders

QUESTIONS

1. Did the phlebotomist violate HIPAA regulations?

2. Did the father have the right to look at his daughter's hospital orders?

3. Did the phlebotomist give the father the correct answer to his question?

DISCUSSION OF CASE STUDY

1. The letters forming the acronym HIPAA refer to the Health Insurance Portability and Accountability Act. This legislation was enacted by Congress in 1996 and was originally established to set standards for the electronic data exchange of medical records information. It has expanded to include many aspects of patient confidentiality. The phlebotomist violated HIPAA regulations by allowing the father to view the physician's orders. Physician's orders are part of the patient's medical record and thus are confidential.

2. The father did not have the right ethically or legally to view his daughter's orders. Patients must give written or verbal consent to have any part of their medical record information revealed to another person, including family members. It is obvious that the father did not know exactly what type of surgery would be performed on his daughter.

3. It does not matter whether the phlebotomist gave the father the correct information or not. It was not her responsibility to explain to a family member or the patient what a test would indicate. She should have directed the father to ask the doctor or the nurse for an explanation. They are qualified to know what information should or should not be given to the patient. Susan also needs to be more careful and to ensure that patient requisitions are not easily viewed by anyone other than those who are allowed to see them.

Quiz

MULTIPLE CHOICE

1. Who can give consent to have blood drawn from a 10-year-old child?
   a. physician
   b. legal guardian
   c. parent
   d. attending nurse
   e. b & c
   f. a & c
   g. b & d

2. Who can give consent and assume liability to have a combative 10-year-old child restrained while his or her blood is drawn by a phlebotomist?
   a. legal guardian
   b. physician
   c. RN
   d. parent
   e. no one
   f. b and c

3. Which of the following would most likely **not** cause a hematoma?
   a. The needle penetrates all the way through the vein.
   b. The needle is only partly inserted into the vein.
   c. The needle is removed after the tourniquet is released.
   d. Excessive blind probing is used to locate the vein.

SELECT THE CORRECT ANSWER FROM CHOICES A TO F.

A. blood-borne pathogen   **D.** reverse isolation

B. airborne isolation   **E.** PPE

C. contact isolation   **F.** nosocomial

4. ___ measles

5. ___ immunocompromised

6. ___ acquired hospital infection

7. ___ vancomycin-resistant *Enterococcus*

8. ___ needle stick injury

9. ___ hepatitis C infection

10. ___ methicillin-resistant *Staphylococcus aureus*

11. ___ mycobacterium TB

12. ___ bone marrow transplantation

13. ___ gloves

FILL IN THE BLANKS.

14. Give three examples of accepted phlebotomy Standard of Care.

_____

_____

_____

When a phlebotomist threatens to hold a patient down if he or she does not cooperate, it is known as _____ in legal terms.

15. If a phlebotomist holds a patient down against his or her will to obtain a blood specimen, it is known as _____ in legal terms.

16. If a phlebotomist leaves a tourniquet on a patient for 10 minutes, it is known as _____ in legal terms.

17. Articles such as gowns, masks, gloves, and syringe transfer devices are commonly called _____.

18. The single most effective means of preventing the spread of infection is_____.

19. Isolation used to prevent the transfer of an organism from one person to another or one object to another is called_____ isolation.

20. N95 mask is used for protection from_____.

21. What are the three components of the Chain of Infection?

    _____ _____ _____

22. The best defense against malpractice is following

    _____ ____ _____ for phlebotomists.

23. Breach of _____ occurs when information about a patient is discussed in a public elevator. This violates the _____ Act.

ESSAY

24. Discuss blood culture contamination, including how it can be reduced and how it can be presented as a quality assurance monitor.

25. Explain with examples how accepted Standard of Care relates to such issues as liability, negligence, assault, battery.

26. Sue discovers a small paper fire in the Laboratory Administration area. What steps, in the correct order, should she take to ensure that the fire is distinguished and all personnel are safe?

    If she used the fire extinguisher, what extinguisher should she use and what steps, in the proper order, should she perform to extinguish the fire?

27. Why is cultural diversity training important? Explain with examples.

28. Discuss why Legal Chain of Custody collection is necessary.

Answers

CHAPTER 1

Question	Answer
1.	e
2.	c
3.	e
4.	a
5.	d
6.	b
7.	d
8.	e
9.	a
10.	c
11.	c
12.	e
13.	d
14.	c
15.	b
16.	b
17.	d
18.	c
19.	e
20.	b
21.	c
22.	a
23.	c

24.	b
25.	d
26.	d
27.	e
28.	e
29.	b
30.	c
31.	e

CHAPTER 2

Question	**Answer**
1.	d
2.	e
3.	d
4.	c
5.	c
6.	d
7.	a
8.	b
9.	a
10.	a
11.	e
12.	c
13.	d
14.	a
15.	b, c, d
16.	c
17.	a
18.	e
19.	e
20.	d
21.	f
22.	F
23.	T

24.	T
25.	F
26.	F
27.	F

CHAPTER 3

Question	Answer
1.	d
2.	e
3.	b
4.	e
5.	a
6.	c
7.	d
8.	d
9.	b
10.	d
11.	b
12.	e
13.	d
14.	d
15.	b
16.	a
17.	e
18.	e
19.	e
20.	e
21.	e
22.	d
23.	c
24.	e
25.	a
26.	d
27.	b

CHAPTER 4

Question	Answer
1.	a
2.	e
3.	b
4.	e
5.	e
6.	d
7.	e
8.	d
9.	b
10.	a
11.	d
12.	e
13.	a
14.	e
15.	e
16.	e
17.	c
18.	b
19.	a
20.	b
21.	e
22.	d
23.	c
24.	b
25.	c
26.	a
27.	d

CHAPTER 5

Question	Answer
1.	e
2.	e
3.	c
4.	b
5.	d
6.	f
7.	c
8.	a
9.	a
10.	c
11.	b
12.	d
13.	f

Glossary

acid-fast bacilli: A particular type of bacterium that will stain red when stained with an acid-fast staining technique. An example is *Mycobacterium tuberculosis*.

allogeneic: In transplantations, from another. Blood or tissue that has similar but not identical antigens is donated by another person.

ammonia: An element within the body that combines weak bonds with acidic compounds and stronger bonds with alkaline compounds. Elevated ammonia levels in the body usually indicate an increased blood urea nitrogen breakdown that is not being eliminated from the body.

antibiotic sensitivity: A drug that can kill or slow down the growth of the organisms.

antibiotic toxicity: The level of drug in a patient that can cause harm to the patient.

anticoagulant: Substance introduced into the blood specimen to keep it from clotting.

anticoagulant-to-blood ratio: A specific volume of anticoagulant to a specific volume of blood.

anti-inflammatory agents: Medicine that aids or prevents inflammation of areas of the body. An example is aspirin.

arteriosclerosis: Blood vessels that supply blood to the heart and brain become hardened because of the interior spaces being clogged by cholesterol plaques.

autoimmune disease: Arising from and directed against the patient's own cells.

autologous: In transplantation, refers to donors who donate their own blood or skin to be transplanted at a later date.

AV shunt: Arteriovenous passage artificially constructed to divert blood flow. Special training is required to draw from this line.

bleeding disorders: Deficiency of coagulation products that can cause excessive patient bleeding (e.g., hemophilia).

bleeding time: Test performed to assess platelet plug formation. The test is often performed before surgery.

blood-borne pathogen: A term applied to any infectious microorganism present in the blood.

blood cultures: A specimen taken from the bloodstream to determine whether organisms are circulating throughout the system; usually timed to coincide with fever. Two cultures are usually taken at specific timed intervals to increase the chances of obtaining the organism(s).

blood pressure: The amount of pressure exerted on a vein.

bone marrow transplantation: Replacement of a patient's own bone marrow with a transplant from a donor. When marrow is defective or cancerous, it can be replaced with healthy blood cells from a donor.

butterfly use: A butterfly is a blood-drawing device used when a vein is small and difficult to draw from. Because using a butterfly instead of a standard Vacutainer method is 5 to 10 times more expensive, care must be taken when deciding to use a butterfly.

cephalic vein: The second-choice vein, located on the lateral side of the arm (thumb side when palms are up) in the antecubital fossa. The vein tends to be smaller, rolls, and is closer to nerves.

Centers for Disease Control and Prevention (CDC): This center is part of the US Public Health Service, which oversees the investigation and control of various diseases, particularly diseases that are communicable and threaten the health of the population.

central venous catheter (CVC): A line inserted into the subclavian vein and advanced into the superior vena cava vein proximal to the right atrium.

chemistry: The study of the chemical properties of a substance and its interactions with other substances.

child abuse: The physical, emotional, or sexual maltreatment of a minor.

chromosome: One of the bodies in the cell nucleus that is the bearer of genes. Humans usually have 46 chromosomes.

cirrhosis: Progressive disease of the liver resulting in damage to and death of hepatic cells, resulting in reduced function of the liver and reduced blood flow, and ultimately, in liver failure.

clotting factors: Elements and compounds necessary for the body to form clots (e.g., Factor 8 and 9, thrombin, fibrin, calcium, etc.).

contact precautions: Precautions used when a patient is infected or colonized with a microorganism that can be transmitted to another patient via person-to-person contact or from a patient care item to another patient.

Coumadin: The brand name of warfarin (sodium warfarin), an anticoagulant that directly inhibits coagulation factor production. A prothrombin time is used to test Coumadin levels.

dehydration: The excess loss of water without immediate replacement.

dermal puncture: Puncturing the skin with a puncture device such as a lancet for the purpose of collecting blood.

diabetes: Metabolic disease in which carbohydrate utilization is reduced because of a deficiency in insulin.

DIC (disseminated intravascular coagulation): Widespread dissemination throughout the blood vessels of tiny microclots. Platelets and clotting factors are decreased, thus clots are present, but the patient is bleeding because of a loss of platelets and clotting factors.

D-dimer: A coagulation test used to determine which fibrin degradation products are present in the blood vessels. Often used when determining the diagnosis of DIC.

diurnal rhythms: Variations in the body's fluids and functions during a 24-hour period. Some hormone levels will change during the day.

discard tube: A tube used to clear a drawing site from possible contamination to the testing specimen. Tube is discarded as a contaminated specimen.

disinfectants: Chemical compounds used to kill microorganisms in work areas.

disorientation: Loss of the sense of familiarity with one's surroundings.

edema: An abnormal accumulation of tissue fluid that might alter test results.

electrolytes: Elements such as potassium and sodium that conduct electricity when in solution. Electrolytes aid in the osmotic balance between elements within the bloodstream and those outside the bloodstream in the tissue.

embryonic stem cells: Stem cells derived from embryos that have the ability to develop into various types of cells in the body.

***Enterococcus* (VRE):** A gram-positive cocco-bacilli that is resistant to the antibiotic vancomycin.

fainting: Loss of consciousness.

fasting: Abstinence from eating or drinking, except water, for approximately 12 to 14 hours before drawing blood.

fibrin: A filamentous protein formed by the interaction of calcium and thrombin with fibrinogen.

fibrin degradation products (FDP): Small fragments of partially digested fibrin found in the bloodstream.

fibrinogen: A protein found in plasma called factor 1, which is essential for coagulation.

Foley catheter: A sterile tube inserted through the urethra into the bladder for the purpose of collecting urine.

gerontology: The specialty concerned with the medical problems and care of older persons.

glucometer: Point-of-care instrument that performs glucose testing at the bedside.

hematology: The study of anatomy, physiology, pathology, etc., related to the blood and blood-forming tissues.

hematoma: A swelling or mass of blood caused by blood leaking from a blood vessel during or after venipuncture.

hematopoietic stem cells: Stem cells that can develop into various types of blood cells.

hemoconcentration: Abnormal concentration of elements and molecules in a confined area. This usually occurs when a tourniquet is left on too long. Values will be falsely elevated.

hemolysis: Destruction of red blood cells, which then release hemoglobin into the liquid portion of the blood. Plasma and serum will appear pink to red. A hemolyzed specimen may give false results because of excess intracellular elements introduced into the fluid.

hemophilia: An inherited disorder of coagulation characterized by a permanent tendency to hemorrhage. Deficiency of factor VIII in the blood coagulation system causes this disorder.

heparin or saline lock: A single-winged needle set that can be left in a patient's vein. Used to draw blood and administer medicine. Special training is required.

hepatitis: Inflammation of the liver from toxic or viral origin. Examples of viral origins are hepatitis B and hepatitis C acquired via unprotected sex, contaminated needles, and blood transfusions.

HIPAC (Hospital Infection Control Practices Advisory Committee): Committee that advises the CDC on updating guidelines regarding prevention of nosocomial infection.

HIV: Human immunodeficiency virus, which causes acquired immunodeficiency syndrome (AIDS).

HIPAA: Health Insurance Portability and Accountability Act, enacted by Congress to protect the confidentiality of electronic transfer of medical record files. It has grown to encompass patient confidentiality throughout health care.

home health care phlebotomy: Phlebotomy performed outside a hospital inside a person's residence. Care must be taken to draw specimens correctly and to transport them safely in the shortest amount of time.

hypertension: High blood pressure.

ice slurry: A combination of ice and water to distribute and maintain an even, cold temperature to keep specimens cold.

immune susceptibility: When a patient's immunity is depressed, thus increasing the chances of infection with a harmful microorganism. The patient's body defenses have been reduced.

implanted port: An implanted vascular device that becomes permanent. Patients can leave the hospital and can come back as outpatients to have their blood drawn from this device. Special training is required.

iron (serum): A metallic element found in hemoglobin, enzymes, etc. Serum iron levels can aid in the diagnosis of iron deficiency anemia.

karyotype: The chromosome characteristics of an individual cell or cell line.

lithium heparin: Anticoagulant used in green-top Vacutainer tubes. The heparin inactivates thrombin to inhibit the coagulation process. Lithium heparin plasma is generally used in the chemistry department.

lumen: The interior space within the vein.

lymphostasis: Obstruction and/or lack of flow of the lymph fluid.

mastectomy: Removal of a breast.

metastatic cancer: Cancer cells that have spread from the original site to another site.

methicillin-resistant *Staphylococcus aureus* (MRSA): Gram-positive organism that is resistant to penicillin-related antibiotics.

mitosis: The usual process of reproduction of cells, consisting of a sequence of modifications of the nucleus that results in the formation of two identical daughter cells with exactly the same chromosome and DNA content as the original cell.

multidrug resistance: Organism is resistant to more than one drug traditionally used to treat the organism.

N95 respirator (category N and 95% efficiency): Respirator used for protection when entering patient rooms with pulmonary tuberculosis or diseases with airborne transmission. Masks are fitted to each employee to guarantee maximum protection.

negative-pressure isolation room: Air circulation and air pressure are designed so that more air comes in than goes out. This decreases the chances of infectious agents being spread to other areas.

negligence: A failure to perform duties according to the standards of the job description.

nerve damage: Inadvertent damage of the nerve by needle stick or pressure on the nerve caused by a hematoma.

newborn screening test: Screening tests performed on newborns to check for the presence of genetic diseases or metabolic disorders that can harm the newborn if not treated.

normal flora: Microorganisms normally existing in a body. In a healthy body they are beneficial, not harmful.

nonadditive tubes: Blood collection tubes without any additive. No clot activator or anticoagulant is present.

obese patient: A patient who is abnormally overweight. An abnormal amount of fat in the arms can increase the difficulty of drawing blood from a patient. Care must be taken that because of the angle of draw the needle does not go through the vein and potentially hit a nerve.

order of draw: The special sequence in which multiple specimen tubes are drawn, designed to reduce the interference of additives between tubes and contamination of tissue thromboplastin.

partial thromboplastin time (PTT): A coagulation test used to test the intrinsic coagulation factors and pathway. This test is usually used when a patient is being treated with heparin.

patient identification: A protocol developed to ensure the proper identification of a patient. For example, the patient could be identified by comparing the name and medical record number from orders and the patient's arm band.

pediatric restraints: Different methods are used to restrain pediatric patients without harming them. For example, wrapping an infant in a blanket or having parents hold down free arms and legs.

petechiae: Pinpoint hemorrhage spots in the skin that may be indicative of a coagulation problem.

personal protective equipment (PPE): Equipment designed to protect health care workers and patients from hazardous substances (i.e., gowns, gloves, goggles, etc.).

pH: Symbol for the H^+ ion concentration within a solution. A pH > 7.0 is alkaline and a ph < 7.0 is acidic.

PKU: Phenylketonuria, an inherited lack of the enzyme to break down the protein phenylalanine. An excess of phenylalanine can produce brain damage that results in mental retardation in infants.

PICC line: Very small vascular access device that is used to give medicine. Blood can be withdrawn from a PICC line, though some departments refuse to draw from this line because too much vacuum will destroy the line.

platelets: Blood cells that aid in the formation of blood clots. It is found in the peripheral blood, is about one-half the size of a red blood cell, and contains no hemoglobin or defined nucleus.

platelet function assay: A precise test to determine the ability to form a platelet plug.

platelet plug: Platelet aggregation and adhesion to an area after an injury plugs up the opening.

point-of-care instrument: Testing device that performs at the bedside, not in the laboratory.

postpartum: After childbirth.

prophylactics: Treatment taken to prevent an infection or disease.

polymerase chain reaction (PCR): A testing method used frequently when testing for viruses.

primary hemostasis: The formation of a platelet plug consisting of platelets only. Secondary hemostasis consists of a plug including platelets, RBCs, and fibrin.

prothrombin time: Prothrombin is a coagulant test used for measuring the extrinsic factors of coagulation. Care must be taken when drawing the specimen to ensure that the blood-to-anticoagulant ratio is 9:1, that the specimen is tested within an acceptable time frame, and that the specimen has not been contaminated.

reverse isolation: Also referred to as protective isolation. Precautions and procedures developed to prevent exposure of a patient to harmful microorganisms. Immunocompromised patients are often placed in reverse isolation.

septicemia: Microorganism(s) circulating in the bloodstream.

sodium citrate: An anticoagulant used for drawing tubes used in coagulation studies.

specimen integrity: The quality of a specimen when received for testing. The specimen should be transported under ideal conditions and have no hemolysis or clot formation.

spleen: A large lymphatic vascular organ existing in the upper part of the left side of the abdominal cavity. It is a blood-forming organ in early life and a storage unit for red blood cells and platelets in later life. The spleen also acts as a blood filter, destroying ineffective red blood cells.

Standard Precautions: A set of infection control safeguards established within an environment to prevent the transmission of microorganisms to others.

therapeutic drug monitoring: Drugs are monitored in a patient to determine the most effective dose to help the patient without causing harm. Trough levels (lowest dose in the body) and peak levels (highest dose in the body) are measured by timed blood draws to determine the level of concentration in the patient's body.

tissue thromboplastin: A substance present in tissue, platelets, and leukocytes necessary for the coagulation of blood. Because of the release of thromboplastin when a needle enters a blood drawing site, the first tube drawn is believed to be contaminated with thromboplastin that may affect coagulation studies performed on that tube.

timed blood draws: Blood draws are timed to monitor the levels of different elements in the body. For example, a hemoglobin and hematocrit sample will be drawn every 4 hours to determine if a patient is actively bleeding or stabilizing.

Vacutainer tubes: Color-coded specimen collection tubes that contain a vacuum so as to aspirate blood when a needle enters a patient's arm.

vancomycin: An antibiotic.

vancomycin-resistant *Enterococcus* **(VRE):** A gram-positive organisms that is resistant to the antibiotic vancomycin.

INDEX

Page numbers in *italics* designate figures; page numbers followed by the letter "t" designate tables; page numbers followed by the letter "b" designate boxes.